PDQ
EVIDENCE-BASED
PRINCIPLES AND
PRACTICE

*PDQ** SERIES

JOHNSON
PDQ PHARMACOLOGY

NORMAN, STREINER
PDQ STATISTICS

STREINER, NORMAN
PDQ EPIDEMIOLOGY

---

*PDQ (Pretty Darned Quick)

PDQ
EVIDENCE-BASED PRINCIPLES AND PRACTICE

ANN McKIBBON, BSc, MLS
Health Information Research Unit
Department of Clinical Epidemiology and Biostatistics
McMaster University
Hamilton, Ontario

with
Angela Eady, BA, MLS and Susan Marks, BA, BEd

1999
B.C. Decker Inc.
Hamilton • London • Saint Louis

B.C. Decker Inc.
4 Hughson Street South
P.O. Box 620, L.C.D. 1
Hamilton, Ontario L8N 3K7
Tel: 905-522-7017; 1-800-568-7281
Fax: 905-522-7839
e-mail: info@bcdecker.com
website: http://www.bcdecker.com

99 00 01 02 / PC / 6 5 4 3 2 1

ISBN 1-55009-118-2

Printed in Canada

Sales and Distribution

United States
B.C. Decker Inc.
P.O. Box 785
Lewiston, NY 14092-0785
Tel: 800-568-7281
e-mail: info@bcdecker.com

Canada
B.C. Decker Inc.
4 Hughson Street South
P.O. Box 620, L.C.D. 1
Hamilton, Ontario L8N 3K7
Tel: 905-522-7017; 800-568-7281
Fax: 905-522-7839
e-mail: info@bcdecker.com

Japan
Igaku-Shoin Ltd.
Foreign Publications Department
3-24-17 Hongo, Bunkyo-ku
Tokyo 113-8719, Japan
Tel: 3 3817 5676; Fax: 3 3815 6776
e-mail: fmbook@ba2.so-net.or.jp

South America
Ernesto Reichmann, Distribuidora de Livros Ltda.
Rua Coronel Marques
335-Tatuape, 03440-000
Sao Paulo-SP-Brazil
Tel/Fax: 011 218 2122

U.K., Europe, Scandinavia, Middle East
Blackwell Science Ltd.
Osney Mead
Oxford OX2 OEL United Kingdom
Tel: 44-1865-206206; Fax: 44-1865-721205
e-mail: blackwell-science.com

Australia
Blackwell Science Asia Pty, Ltd.
54 University Street
Carlton, Victoria 3053
Australia
Tel: 03 9347 0300
Fax: 03 9347 5001
e-mail: info@blacksci-asia.com.au

Korea
Seoul Medical Scientific Books Co.
C.P.O. Box 9794
Seoul 100 697
South Korea
Tel: 82 2925 5800
Fax: 82 2927 7283

Foreign Rights
John Scott & Co.
International Publishers' Agency
P.O. Box 878
Kimberton, PA 19442
Tel: 610-827-1640
Fax: 610-827-1671

To George

Contents

Foreword

With over 50 years of increasingly robust biomedical research since the end of World War II, and a worldwide investment of over $50 billion in new research each year, it is hardly astonishing that health care practitioners and patients are having a tough time keeping on top of the new knowledge. Textbooks, the traditional first resort for clinical queries, are inadequate to the task for a number of reasons. First, textbooks are published on what are now lengthy cycles compared with the advance of knowledge, typically with 3 or more years between editions. Second, textbook authors either have limited knowledge of what constitutes sound evidence for clinical practice, or override (inadvertently, one presumes) sound evidence with their "expertise". Third, the biomedical literature is too poorly organized at present for reliable, easy access to best evidence on a given clinical topic.

These limitations of evidence-based services for clinical decisions are under assault through advances in information access and improved standards for reporting, sorting, distilling, synthesizing, disseminating, and integrating new evidence into health care decisions. But these innovations are far from mature and themselves outstrip the abilities of practitioners and patients to understand and properly use them. Clinicians and patients need help if patients are to receive current best care—*your* health care provider needs help if *you* are to receive current best care, should you need medical attention.

The most important messages of this book are that you can help health care providers do their jobs, and help patients to understand their problems so that they can be more effective partners in their own care. Most care for complex health disorders requires multidisciplinary teamwork, the more so as the population ages and people accumulate numerous ills. Information specialists should be regular members of the team, facilitating access to best sources of information for the questions that frequently arise in practice, and forwarding new information as it becomes available. Of course, there are not enough information specialists to fill such roles, and there is limited appreciation at present that "informologists" are needed to help save lives and reduce suffering. So the challenges for information specialists become to work as efficiently as possible to meet the requests they currently receive, to build better information services for the future, and to teach health professionals to become proficient themselves in evaluating and applying evidence-based information services.

This book contains the knowledge and wisdom that health professionals will need to participate as collaborators in the information revolution as it applies to supporting evidence-based health care. Written by one of my heroes, Ann McKibbon, it takes readers through the basic principles of what constitutes best evidence for health care practice and how it can be quickly found, using modern information facilities. Rich with current examples and illustrations of how evidence can be matched with clinical information needs, I believe it will provide a stellar resource for all who desire to improve the orderly transfer of knowledge into practice in the health sciences.

And why is Ann McKibbon my hero, you ask? I've worked with Ann for over a decade since she responded to an advertisement for a position as a research librarian. She has been a leader in our health informatics team since then, developing and evaluating innovations that might improve the match between what is known from sound research and what practitioners know and apply when they offer care to patients. During that time, Ann has taught me more about information services than I would have imagined possible. She is an expert (in the best sense of the word) in information science and an influential educator, with a worldwide reputation for her research and teaching. At last, with urging from many fans, she has put pen to paper to summarize her knowledge.

Readers are in for a treat! The secrets of evidence-based health information are revealed here. Those who learn them will be able to help health practitioners take better care of their patients, and people take better care of their own health. What better way to avert the tragedy of people languishing "in the midst of plenty" because they and their clinical providers lack best evidence that can be, and ought to be, at their fingertips or quickly available on request?

R. Brian Haynes, MD, PhD
Professor of Clinical Epidemiology and Medicine
McMaster University
Hamilton, Ontario, Canada

Preface

My exposure to evidence-based health care (EBHC) principles started in the late 1970s before the term was coined. My job was part-time, temporary, and irregular for three months, preparing an evidence-based annotated bibliography of the literature of continuing medical education. I was the only librarian working with a committee of physicians and administrators who were trying to evaluate the literature to understand how health professionals learn and keep up-to-date after they graduate. The committee members were from the Department of Clinical Epidemiology and Biostatistics at McMaster University, and the continuing medical education project was part of the development of the ideas and principles of critical appraisal and EBHC.

Although initially the concepts seemed complex and encumbered by a large amount of jargon, I found the principles interesting and intellectually challenging, yet firmly based on common sense and reason. Over the past 20 years I have worked with, taught and learned from, and enjoyed being with clinicians, epidemiologists, statisticians, and librarians at McMaster University and in the broader health care community. During that time I have become convinced that EBHC is a rich and essential foundation for all aspects of health care.

Cindy Walker Dilks and I have taught more than 50 courses on three continents on EBHC and information retrieval: the material covered in this book. Initially audiences comprised librarians working in large academic libraries in universities and teaching hospitals, but many more groups of health professionals want to improve their information retrieval skills. We can no longer keep up with the demand for individual workshops. The impetus for this book has grown from the class notes of the workshops and our desire to present the course material more fully than we are able to in an eight-hour class. We have designed the book for anyone who wants to understand the building blocks and conceptual underpinnings of the process of EBHC and wants to develop strong information retrieval skills. This book is useful to both professionals and those making health care decisions for themselves, and assisting with decision making for their families, and friends.

OBJECTIVES

This book and CD-ROM are meant to be a stand-alone pair of documents. The two major objectives are, first, for readers to improve their abilities to understand the process of EBHC and the theoretical basis of health care research; and second, to effectively and efficiently retrieve material of value in making clinical decisions. The total body of biomedical research literature has many purposes—such as communication among researchers, and among researchers and clinicians—but appropriate information or evidence for clinical decisions makes up only one small segment of the whole literature. Because application of published evidence is a vital part of the EBHC process, and the literature that is ready for clinical application is a small segment of the total volume of health care literature, learning how to retrieve material quickly and efficiently is essential. Secondary objectives of the book are:

1. To offer the reader an understanding of the historical basis and current practice of health care research: that is that part of biological or basic research that is clinically relevant or ready for clinical application. This includes understanding basic research methodology for therapy, diagnosis, etiology and causation, natural history and prognosis, economics, and qualitative studies, along with secondary publications such as systematic reviews and clinical practice guidelines.

2. To review how original studies and systematic review articles in each of the content areas are indexed by MEDLINE, CINAHL, EMBASE, and PsycINFO. These four bibliographic databases are the major sources of literature or evidence used by most clinicians who apply published evidence in their decision-making. MEDLINE is produced by the U.S. National Library of Medicine and covers all areas of health care research, with strengths in basic science and clinical medicine. It includes more than 9 million citations from 1966, which were published in more than 4,000 journals. CINAHL (Cumulative Index to Nursing and Allied Health Literature) is a commercial product that provides coverage of allied health care literature, with strengths in nursing, physiotherapy, occupational therapy, alternative therapies, and other related areas. It is a smaller but richer database than MEDLINE; it includes more than basic citations to journal articles. It also contains bibliographies of cited articles, theses, technical reports, full-text clinical practice guidelines, and other related items. PsycINFO is the computer equivalent of *Psychological Abstracts*, and is produced by the American Psychological Association. It provides coverage of psychology, psychiatry, counseling, and other topics related to mental health. EMBASE/Excerpta Medica is considered by many to be the European equivalent of MEDLINE. It is a large database and has strengths in pharmacologic literature, allied health areas, and, especially, European literature. As part of accomplishing our second objective we will learn which terms indexers of these four databases have available for indexing each category of original and review research, and examine the terms and phrases authors of the study reports use in their titles and abstracts. More information on each of these databases and other information sources is available in Chapter 1.

3. To give experience in retrieving these clinically relevant studies from the four databases. Searching examples will be provided which show both the power and problems with "methodology-based" retrievals for original and systematic review articles.

4. To introduce some of the basic statistical techniques used in studies in various categories. Examples are included in each chapter, so that readers can calculate basic statistics for therapy and diagnosis studies and appreciate how statistics from other categories are calculated and presented.

CONTENT

This book covers most of the material and topics that are included in basic, university-level clinical epidemiology courses. It also includes examples of research studies, how authors present the results of their studies, and how indexers from the four databases index them. The book is part of the *PDQ* series, and is therefore designed to include some aspects of a workbook. The theoretical principles are supplemented with many real and hypothetical examples from all disciplines of health care. The searching assignments at the end of each chapter have suggested solutions in the CD-ROM appendix. The research basis, or evidence, on which the book is based is a study by Haynes et al.[1] that formally evaluates the retrievals of search strategies designed to retrieve citations of only clinically relevant studies. The study is described more fully in the therapy and diagnosis chapters. Study funding came from the U.S. National Library of Medicine and the Ontario Ministry of Health.

ACKNOWLEDGMENTS

This book would not have been possible without my friends and colleagues in the Health Information Research Unit of the Department of Clinical Epidemiology and Biostatistics at McMaster University: Cindy Walker Dilks, Brian Haynes, Nancy Wilczynski, Susan Marks, Angela Eady, and Dawn Jedras. Special thanks also goes to a special group of clinicians who have inspired and challenged me to new and broader ways of thinking and acting—Mike Zaroukian, Bob McNutt, Larry Blonde, Alex Jadad, Pat Brill Edwards, Dereck Hunt, Alba DiCenso, Donna Ciliska, Nicky Cullum, Roman Jaeschke, Scott Richardson, Mark Wilson, and Rosanne Leipzig. Health sciences librarians in Hamilton and throughout North America have also been invaluable in the evolution of this book. Several deserve special thanks: Liz Bayley was always there when I needed her, Katy Nesbit provided the CINAHL searching terms and phrases, and Jean Sullivant provided the same for PsycINFO; Rose Marie Woodsmall and Anna Harbourt have shown and taught me much—the rest are too numerous to mention, but you know who you are. Thanks to all of you.

REFERENCE

1. Haynes RB, Wilczynski NL, McKibbon KA, et al. Developing optimal search strategies for detecting clinically sound studies in MEDLINE. J Am Med Inform Assoc 1994;1:447–58.

Introduction

The reality of the information explosion is something health care professionals and librarians deal with daily. Technology, software, and the Internet give us the impression that the explosion is actually gaining in force and magnitude. A major motivation for the development of online databases such as MEDLINE, and the Internet itself, was to have better control of literature and information. This motivation remains only partly realized, because we do not necessarily have better control; we just have faster access to more information. These are exciting times for anyone who is interested in information access. New tools and skills are being developed, and more are needed for us to rise to these information processing challenges.

Health care professionals cannot rely for long on the information and skills they have learned by the time they graduate. An approach to the practice of health care called **evidence-based medicine** has become formalized and advocated in the past decade.[1–3] Although many clinicians have always practiced this way, the formalization of the processes has made evidence-based medicine more visible, more desirable, and easier to implement. A large component of this movement includes harnessing and using the health care literature as the basis for practice decisions in conjunction with clinical experience, strong basic education, and the patient's unique situation. Although medicine was one of the first disciplines to adopt evidence-based medicine principles, other health care disciplines have also adopted the principles and processes. The practices of evidence-based nursing, evidence-based mental health, evidence-based dentistry, evidence-based cardiology, and even evidence-based podiatry and evidence-based bone and joint surgery have been recognized in the literature. General overall terms of evidence-based practice or evidence-based health care have been suggested to cover discussions of all disciplines. This book will use the general term *evidence-based health care* (EBHC) unless a specific discipline is discussed. The terms "clinician" and "health care professional" will be used to encompass all those who help patients and families make appropriate health care and related decisions: physicians, nurses, dentists, clergy, physio-and occupational therapists, psychologists, midwives, and so on.

EVIDENCE-BASED HEALTH CARE DEFINITION

Evidence-based health care is a process of health care decision-making and related behavior. Several definitions have been developed to describe it. Definition one[1] states that clinicians who practice EBHC build on their clinical experience and formal education (knowledge of pathophysiology and mechanisms of action) using current evidence from the published literature. Experience and basic knowledge are necessary, but not sufficient, for the practice of EBHC. Clinicians need to ground their practice in fundamental principles and then base their decisions and actions on appropriate evidence from health care research, taking into account the unique needs of the patient. This evidence can be from either original studies or trials or evidence-based secondary sources, such as systematic review articles and meta-analyses, decision analysis tools, clinical practice guidelines, and economic analyses. Definition one also emphasizes that knowing how to use the literature is imperative for ensuring that clinicians are providing optimal care.

According to definition two, EBHC[2] "is the process of systematically finding, appraising, and using contemporaneous research findings as the basis for clinical decisions." The key idea here is use of research findings that are currently the best available. Evidence-based health care means a strong commitment to keeping up-to-date with changing and improving health care innovations that are reported in the literature.

What is lacking, or at least not explicit in these first two definitions, is that the patient involved in the decision must be recognized as having his or her own needs, expectations, culture, spiritual beliefs, and preferences, and should take part in the decision-making process. The clinical setting, resources, practical implications, and cost constraints must also be considered on a case-by-case basis.

Definition three is the one most often used in describing EBHC.[3] It reads: "... the conscientious, explicit, and judicious use of current best evidence in making decisions about the care of individual patients." The definition implies conscious choice on the part of the clinician and patient, explicit and exact decisions being made and carried out, and always wisdom, experience, and judgment used to evaluate and apply this evidence. An individual patient with a specific need or problem is almost always involved. This definition reinforces and recognizes that EBHC is really the way many feel that our best clinicians have always practiced.

FIVE STEPS OF EVIDENCE-BASED HEALTH CARE

Evidence-based health care is actually a five-step process, and each step takes time and energy. All five steps can take up to an hour or longer to complete, depending on the complexities and access to the original studies. The first step is defining the question that needs to be answered: this is often more difficult than first envisioned. Librarians often equate this step with the "reference interview" process that takes place each time a person asks for library assistance. The second step is collecting evidence to answer the question. This is the step where librarians can (and should) play a key role. This role can involve the provision of the evidence itself, or teaching clinicians and clinicians-in-training how to effectively and efficiently find evidence in the health care literature. The third and fourth steps are the ones that utilize basic knowledge and previous clinical experience. Third is the formal evaluation of the evidence gathered. This step is also called **critical appraisal**—the reading and analysis of the studies found, taking into account the patient, setting, situation, and problem as defined. Fourth is the integration of the evidence and patient factors to make and carry out the decision. The fifth step, one often omitted, is the evaluation of the whole process with a view to improving it the next time the EBHC cycle is followed.

Clinicians who use EBHC techniques do not use the five steps for every one of their health care encounters. Often the full five-step process is done once or twice a week on a specific question that the clinician feels needs consideration. An example of this would be a general internist who has noticed several new studies of drugs for congestive heart failure. At home one evening she mentally reviews the three patients she has seen that day, and is worried about one patient who does not seem to be responding to the usual drug regimen. She wonders if she should change or update her prescribing for Mr. Augustine for his congestive heart failure which is complicated by insulin-dependent diabetes mellitus. She determines the question she wishes to address, does a literature search, reads two articles, and decides that Mr. Augustine does not need to start amiodarone therapy. Because of this review of new drugs for congestive heart failure she has confirmed that how she cares for these patients is current and appropriate. As this pattern of several EBHC cycles per week is followed, most of the common situations a clinician encounters will be addressed and updated, if needed. Clinicians can never be completely current, especially when patients present with diseases or conditions that are uncommon in their practice. Evidence-based health care "allows" that clinicians cannot know or be current on everything, and provides mechanisms for helping them give the best care they can. In addition, good clinicians know their own abilities and when to treat or refer patients.

CRITICISMS

As with any new development, EBHC has its detractors. Criticisms need to be evaluated to ascertain if refinements or improvements are needed. Much wisdom and understanding is often gained by a thorough and honest evaluation of others reactions and comments. *The Lancet* editors[4] accused EBHC proponents of being subversive, narrow, and lacking finesse, with the "movement" having certain similarities to fundamentalist cults.

Any new movement always has individuals who are excited and want to change standard behavior and practice. In addition, movements often start with a simplistic "black-white" view of reality which matures and becomes more complex as features of the movement become incorporated into routine use. If these two features of EBHC are true, then *The Lancet* editors are probably right in their assessment. EBHC will however er grow and mature as it becomes incorporated into the fabric of health care.

In a more gentle but substantive critique, Feinstein and Horowitz[5] point out that the "laudable goal of making clinical decisions based on evidence" must be tempered by three additional truths. The first, and probably most important, is that each patient brings his or her own situation, preferences, culture, and needs, all of which must be balanced with the evidence. Second, today's golden truth may easily be tomorrow's inaccurate, or even inappropriate, information. Finally, many of our current best-care practices have not, nor ever will be, evaluated using the best of EBHC approaches. There are several reasons for this absence of evaluation. Ethics do not allow researchers to withhold blood transfusions from accident victims to test if the transfusions will save lives, or refuse to give fluids to young infants who are dehydrated merely for testing purposes. Common sense tells us that children should wear mittens when they go out in the snow, even though this has not been formally studied. Funding agencies are not interested in financing large-scale studies on topics such as the removal of ear wax. Other examples of these "gray areas" of practices that are not solidly evaluated are the use of some antibiotics for infections, antidepressants for depression, implantable pacemakers for symptomatic heart block, and catheterization for urinary obstruction.

COMMUNICATION AND RESEARCH

The rest of this chapter gives the historic background of biomedical communication and research. The book then describes how current biomedical research is conducted, reported, and used by health professionals. Six major primary clinical research types are studied: therapy, diagnosis, etiology and causation, prognosis and natural history, economics, and qualitative research (the understanding of the processes of disease and health). The basic methodologies unique to each research type, along with examples of good and bad research are provided. The secondary EBHC literature (systematic review articles and clinical practice guidelines) are also studied. Information is also given on how indexers index articles of each type of research, and how this indexing can be used along with abstract and title words to retrieve ready-for-clinical-application material.

A combination of approaches for each research area is used to develop methodological filters for MEDLINE, CINAHL, PsycINFO, and EMBASE searching using clinical examples. When to use this methodological filtering is discussed, and sample questions are included at the end of each chapter. The appendix in the CD-ROM includes several proposed answers from various databases for each clinical question. Also described are several EBHC products, such as *Best Evidence* from the American College of Physicians—American Society of Internal Medicine and the *BMJ* Publishing Group, and the *Cochrane Library* from the Cochrane Collaboration and Update Software. Your feedback is valued. Please send us any hints or techniques you discover in your work with EBHC.

HISTORY OF SCIENTIFIC COMMUNICATION

Evidence-based health care has its roots in ancient history. Men and women have always strived to learn, experiment, and pass on their knowledge and experience. To properly understand the current state of health care research, one needs to start with a review of the historic process of scientific communication and its various stages of development.

ORAL TRADITION

Story-telling and the oral tradition were the first methods used to communicate, teach, and pass on knowledge and skills. Story-telling was the main form of scientific communication for many centuries. The oral tradition for transfer of health care information is still used in many cultures today, either formally through village healers in less-developed countries, or through the handing-down of home or folk remedies from one generation to another. Oral communication of health care information is still used in current care situations such as morning report, case presentations, and patient history taking. Formal communication of scientific ideas however is no longer oral-based.

LETTERS

Writing developed 5,000 years ago,[6] and several centuries later the Greeks and Romans started to write letters to each other. Scientific communication was probably not the first use of letter writing, but it was not long before letters were routinely exchanged by philosophers, mathematicians, and other thinkers. Archimedes and Ptolemy were among the first to write to their friends and acquaintances, telling them of their scientific ideas and theories. Letters began formal, recorded modes of scientific communication, and this continued for many centuries.

HANDWRITTEN BOOKS

Handwritten letters soon evolved into handwritten books. These were very valuable to the few people who could read them. Handwritten books were scarce because they were difficult to reproduce. The library in ancient Alexandria was legendary for its collection of medical texts, and when it was destroyed much knowledge was lost. Copies of medical texts were kept by the monasteries, and they were often tended with as much care as the religious texts.

PRINTING PRESS AND BOOKS

The next major advance in scientific communication was the development of the printing press more than 500 years ago in Germany. The first mass-produced books, like the handwritten ones, were in Latin, the language of the clerics and the intelligentsia. The first illustrated medical textbook was printed in 1495[7] and a recent issue of *JAMA* has reproduced several wood cuts from the text. Johannes de Ketham was the author of *Fasciculus Medicine* which was printed in Venice. It included descriptions of various common diagnostic and therapeutic procedures such as blood letting, urine examination, pregnancy care, and behavior during epidemics. As more books became available and education spread to the masses, books were written in the common language. Several centuries after the development of the printing press, mass-produced books became the major vehicle for scientific communication.

GUILD SYSTEM AND JOURNALS

In the 1600s the guild system became part of the fabric of industry, technology, and science. Scientists established their own societies and soon started writing short communications for presentation at society meetings. These short pieces were subsequently printed in new publications such as *Philosophical Transactions* and *Transactions of the Royal Society of London*. These collections of short presentations became the first journals. Not all scientists, however, agreed that the new journals were a scientific advancement. Sir Isaac Newton felt that these new journal articles lacked propriety, and would have nothing to do with them. He felt persons who did not have enough thoughts, ideas, and facts to fill a book did not deserve to be called scientists. Sir Isaac is buried near the altar in Westminster Cathedral. A large marble statue shows him reclining in a toga, supported by several large books—still preferring them to journals.

However, by the eighteenth century journal articles had become the most widely used scientific communication method.[8] As journals spread, books provided less *new* information and became tools that integrated knowledge: the textbooks, handbooks, and encyclopedias we have today.

PRINTED INDEXES

Two hundred years later, modern biomedical researchers and health care professionals still rely on journal articles for communication of ideas and advancements. Because of the quantity published, persons who use journal literature also must use indexes, both paper and online, to help them find information. Indexing and abstracting services such as *Index Medicus* and *Chemical Abstracts*, were developed approximately 100 years ago, when the number of journals grew so large that formal indexing systems were required to determine what had been published and where. *Index Medicus*, developed by a U.S. surgeon named John Shaw Billings, was one of the first indexes of the medical literature, with many more, such as *Excerpta Medica* and *Psychological Abstracts* being developed in later years. *Cumulative Index to Nursing and Allied Health Literature* was started by the early 1940s to index the nursing literature and the original three-by-five-inch card file which was the basis of the index still exists.

COMPUTER DATABASES

Computerized versions of these indexes were developed starting in the late 1960s. Computer tapes of the bibliographic information were first made to speed the publication of printed indexes. It was not long, however, until developers realized that the computer tapes used in typesetting could be harnessed to provide searching capabilities. The online versions were necessary because of the large numbers of new journals and scientific papers being produced. Early computerized retrieval searching systems were often batch mode processes that required long turnaround times. Teletype machines with paper tape output and acoustic couplers were one of the next advances in the early days of online searching. The staff at the National Library of Medicine required that searchers pass a 4-month training course in MEDLINE search techniques before they were certified and allowed to search. This was soon reduced to a 2–4 week course. Mandatory training was still enforced well into the 1980s. Initially only librarians did online searching, but with the proliferation of computers and telecommunication networks in the late 1980s and early 1990s, anyone with the right equipment can and does use these systems. In fact, my 15-year-old daughter was asked to go on the Internet and use MEDLINE to find some disease-related material in a tenth grade biology class assignment. All of the students in the class finished the routine assignment with no major problems.

THE INTERNET

The Internet has given both health professionals and the lay public almost instantaneous access to enormous amounts of information. The Internet has tremendous implications for EBHC. The large volume is potentially beneficial but much of it is not organized well. The editor of *Scientific American*, in a special issue devoted to the Internet, sums up what all librarians have known for a long time.

"…And so, at some point, the Internet has to stop looking like the world's largest rummage sale. For taming this particular frontier, the right people *are* librarians, not the cowboys. The Internet is made of information, and nobody knows more about how to order information than librarians, who have been pondering that problem for thousands of years."[9]

Much health care information is available with many new publications becoming available online, either duplicating hard copies or in online format alone. The quality of the information is difficult to evaluate and the peer review process that evaluates journal articles is not enforced. The Internet is, however, here to stay, but wisdom and skill are needed to use it effectively, evaluate the quality and usefulness of the information and learn how to deal wisely and appropriately with a proportion of the lay public who are sophisticated users of health care information. More research and understanding is needed on many fronts.

In summary, most scientific communication is still done using journal articles, but because of the quantity and varied formats of published health care information, using health care research requires indexes, online computer systems, and, increasingly, the Internet. The size and complexity of the literature means it is difficult to retrieve citations relevant to the content of the question and appropriate for clinical decision-making. Easy, fast, and efficient retrieval skills can be developed, however, if one understands how the health care literature is structured.

PUBLISHING WEDGE

The biomedical literature is hierarchical in nature, and includes many types or categories of journal articles. Figure 1–1 shows these categories and how they fit into a publishing and research hierarchy of seven levels. Biomedical researchers and clinicians must use material from all seven levels in their area of study, although the researchers often specialize in material from one level or another. To illustrate this, imagine a basic researcher who works on an animal model for a specific disease, such as scabies in sheep: a look-alike disease for multiple sclerosis. This researcher can concentrate on literature published in a narrow range of categories of information. Clinicians, on the other hand, need to use information on treatments for many diseases or conditions, some of which have been firmly and convincingly proved, and some less certain as a basis for clinical decision-making.

The publishing wedge for therapy depicted in Figure 1–1 represents the structure of the health care literature that evaluates interventions. It shows both the types of publication and their relative numbers. All levels on the wedge are important to the process of discovering and proving health care treatment advances, but not all levels are equally useful for making patient care decisions. Other, similar wedges could be drawn for health care research into the areas of diagnostic and screening test evaluation, etiology and causation studies, prognosis and natural history questions, and economic analysis, and for secondary publications.

From the top of the wedge, where numerous "ideas" papers exist, we move through a series of levels to the relatively few that report on ready-for-application clinical

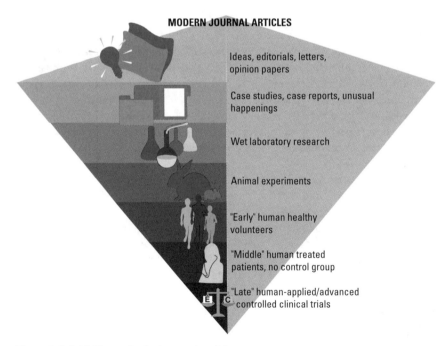

MODERN JOURNAL ARTICLES

Ideas, editorials, letters, opinion papers

Case studies, case reports, unusual happenings

Wet laboratory research

Animal experiments

"Early" human healthy volunteers

"Middle" human treated patients, no control group

"Late" human-applied/advanced controlled clinical trials

Figure 1–1 Publishing wedge for intervention trials.

research (the ones that are appropriate for EBHC decision making). The number of publications in each level decreases substantially, with, it is hoped only the best from each level moving on to the next step.

Level 1: "Ideas" Papers

The first level in the publishing wedge includes "ideas" papers. Many are published, in the health literature; they include such items as editorials, letters to the editor, and general "think" pieces. One example of an ideas paper is that by T.C. Britton.[9] He tries to come to grips with people who have dysfunctional handwriting after stroke and other neurological disease. He describes his thoughts using the terms *dysgraphia*, *agraphia*, and *hypergraphia*. Dysfunctional writing after strokes is distressing and it must be understood before it can be modified or improved.

Level 2: Case Reports

At the next broad level, ideas are discussed in relation to one or several patients: reports of single or of a few cases (case studies), or of unusual happenings. The conclusions or assumptions made on the basis of these papers are often later rejected, but they are the papers we remember. Two examples that stand out in my memory are "blue jeans thighs" occurring when children with new, unwashed blue jeans, wet diapers, and discolored legs are brought to the emergency department by distraught parents;[11] and a case of pulmonary embolism in a hockey player after ingesting the fumes from the Zamboni ice cleaning machine.[12] Now hockey players and ice dancers have their very own disorder—Zamboni disease. A more serious example is one that looks at the potential danger of scurvy caused by malnutrition in patients who have cancer.[13] Fain and colleagues describe six men who were diagnosed with scurvy from 1993 to 1996 among 3723 patients with cancer. All improved after they were given vitamin C. Because of this case report, clinicians who treat patients with cancer can be aware that this potentially serious disease can occur, and become vigilant for indications of scurvy.

Level 3: Laboratory Testing

Some of the ideas from the previous section or level will go on to wet laboratory testing: the test-tube-and-beaker stage. As with all levels, information and knowledge gained while evaluating the ideas in this level (the laboratory) are essential in health care research. If information from levels further down the wedge is, however, available, it is not the information that physicians and nurses should be using in making patient care decisions. The paper by Galimand et al., for example, describes a laboratory study of plasma from a young boy from Madagascar who had had the plague.[14] The laboratory personnel were not interested in finding ways to cure and care for him (that had already happened), but were interested in how drug-resistant *Yersina pestis* isolates reacted to various standard antibiotics.

Level 4: Animal Experiments

Promising findings from the laboratory level are passed on to the next step in the evaluation process: animal experimentation. Not everyone agrees with using animals in research, but modern health care would be poorer without it. As an example of a study from this level, Muhlestein and colleagues are building on research that comes from the knowledge that peptic ulcers are caused by infection with *Helicobacter pylori* bacteria. This has completely changed the practice of gastroenterology. Some new evidence shows that atherosclerosis may be caused by infection with *Chlamydia pneumoniae*.[15] If atherosclerosis is caused by a bacterium, cardiologists will need to make substantial changes in their management of their patients. Muhlestein et al. studied rabbits and infected them with *C. pneumoniae* to ascertain if the infection causes atherosclerosis, and if it does, whether treatment with antibiotics either retards progression of atherosclerosis or reduces it. The current research is still far from clinical application but is moving along in the evaluation process.

Level 5: Early Human Experiments (Phase I Trials)

Three levels of the research wedge for therapies are devoted to evaluation in humans. Evaluations from the first level (also know as Phase I trials) use a limited number of humans, usually volunteers, often in the range of 5 to 15 individuals and last only a short time. Researchers evaluate drugs or other interventions for obvious adverse effects. Marcurad et al.[16] studied healthy volunteers who were evaluated for their absorption of vitamin B_{12} after taking omeprazole. The men studied had no clinical need to take the omeprazole, but researchers wanted to know about potential adverse effects. A general rule of thumb is that Phase I trials take a year to plan, execute, and complete. Again, information proved at this point is important to the whole research and evaluation process, but the clinical usefulness of the information is still limited.

Level 6: Case Series (Phase II Trials)

The second human therapy testing level is known as the Phase II trials. In these studies, researchers often treat a small series of consecutive or carefully selected patients with a new drug or other intervention such as surgery, counseling, or physical exercise programs. Often, no control or comparison group is included. An example of a study from this level of publication is one by Schumacher et al.[17] They evaluated 20 consecutive patients who were scheduled for triple coronary bypass surgery. When the grafting was done, a small amount of human growth factor was injected around the new vein to ascertain if the growth factor, an expensive drug, would help establish new capillaries and improve or speed return of cardiac function. After some time, more new capillaries than expected had grown around the graft in most patients. If this advance continues to show promise in the research process to improve coronary care, many persons will likely benefit. Phase II trials generally take two years from start to finish.

Sildenafil, or Viagra, was first developed as a antihypertensive agent; and it was at this Phase II stage of testing that researchers felt that the high blood pressure was not being lowered effectively, and they chose to stop evaluating this drug for hypertension. The women in the study returned their unused medication as asked, but the men refused because of the side effects they had been experiencing. After questioning them, researchers decided that sildenafil had other marketing possibilities, and the progression through the research wedge was recommenced this time evaluating sildenafil for its ability to treat sexual dysfunction in men.

Level 7: Cinical Trials (Phase III Trials)

The third level (Phase III trials) comprises the studies that EBHC practitioners advocate all health care professionals use in making patient care decisions. These trials are often large and very labor- and resource-intensive. They are the ones, however, that have enough "power" and design strength to separate true health care advances from those that produce more harm than good. The CLASP trial[18] was designed to answer the question of whether aspirin protects pregnant women with hypertension and their infants from the morbidity and mortality associated with pre-eclampsia and eclampsia. Both of these conditions are significant problems in the developed world. Data from all six levels of the research wedge suggested that aspirin was a simple, effective, and low-cost treatment that could save lives and improve maternal and infant outcomes such as seizures in the mother and low birth weight and intrauterine growth retardation in the infant. In the CLASP trial 9362 pregnant women were studied; half received aspirin, 60 mg per day, and half received placebo. When the data were analyzed, outcomes for women allocated to aspirin were shown to be equivalent to the outcomes for women who received placebo. Calcium was also thought to be an important agent to improve maternal and infant health in pre-eclampsia and eclampsia. It, too, was shown to be ineffective in the large clinical trial (at the point of the wedge). Women at risk for blood pressure problems in pregnancy are not routinely given aspirin or calcium to prevent pre-eclampsia and its related problems, based on these two large studies. Phase III trials often take a minimum of three years to complete, and require at least several hundreds of thousands of dollars to fund.

Phase IV Trials

Phase IV trials are "beyond the point of the wedge," and are often called post-marketing studies. They are designed to evaluate the long-term safety and rare adverse effects, and sometimes the economics of drugs or interventions that have already been proved useful in Phase III trials. Long-term safety aspects are discussed in the therapy chapter, adverse effects in the etiology and causation chapter, and economics has its own chapter.

Summary of Wedge

The discussion of the "intervention" wedge includes areas of therapy or treatment (for example, can I use antibiotics for recurrent otitis media?), quality improvement (for example, will a computer-generated reminder increase the rate of signed advance directives by elderly patients?), and prevention and control (for example, how can I keep coronary vessels free of restenosis after successful thrombolysis and angioplasty?). Besides the intervention wedge, wedges also exist for diagnostic or screening studies (for example, can we find a simple blood test to predict which patients in the emergency department with chest pain are having a myocardial infarction, so that those who need treatment receive it and those who are not having a myocardial infarction are evaluated correctly, reassured, and sent home; or, should we screen all adults for colorectal cancer using fecal occult blood tests?). A wedge also exists for etiology and causation studies (for example, what lifestyle factors predispose a person to, or protect them from, developing Alzheimer's disease?); and for prognosis and natural history (for example, what is the natural grieving process after a miscarriage, and what factors, if any, predict which women may need extra support to come to terms with the loss?).

Only one idea in 5000 makes it through the testing for most areas of health care and becomes available for clinical application.[19] In some areas of health care, such as cancer drugs, the numbers are even greater. More than 40,000 potential drugs start at the top of the wedge to find, evaluate, and prove one effective cancer medication. Therefore, effective retrieval skills are vital for health care decision making. This book concentrates on understanding clinical trials and other study designs that form the body of evidence that EBHC practitioners advocate for use in making decisions (material at the point of the evidence wedges) and how they can be retrieved for application.

Not all areas of health care have been studied and evaluated down to this final level. When evidence does exist at this point of the wedge, clinicians should use it in patient care. Conversely, when evidence does not exist at the point of the wedge, as is often the case, EBHC dictates that evidence from the level closest to the point of the wedge should be used.

INFORMATION NEEDS OF RESEARCHERS AND CLINICIANS

Biomedical researchers should know all, or at least most, of the literature in their fields. Their grants, jobs, and reputations demand this. Fortunately, these researchers can often focus on a very specialized and narrow range of topics. Because of this narrowness, their task is not quite as daunting as it seems. In addition, their jobs encourage and allow them time for reading. More important, however, because they are generally located at academic institutions, researchers have good access to the needed information and library resources.

Health care professionals, in contrast to biomedical researchers, must know about a broad range of topics (albeit to a lesser depth). This is especially true if they are generalists rather than specialists such as family physicians rather than cardiovascular surgeons. They also have less time to read, and often do not have the library resources and services that are available to the research community.

RESOURCES FOR CLINICAL STUDIES

It would be fairly simple for health care professionals to keep up-to-date if easy access to current best evidence for patient care existed in one source. Journals that publish only reports of advanced tip-of-the-wedge research involving patients who are similar to their own *do not exist!* Even core clinical journals defined by the U.S. National Library of Medicine (those 125 journals that they feel cover the major advances in clinical care) and those on recommended health care journals lists include articles from all levels of research, and include editorials, letters, professional news, and articles of a broad general nature—none of which reliably support good patient care.

A clinician needs information from five different information sources to provide high-quality and up-to-date care. We will discuss each of these five sources and the types of information they provide, give examples of specific evidence-based resources for each source and describe how they can be accessed or obtained, and provide some initial start-up tips and techniques to get the maximum out of each resource. The five sources are: textbooks (repositories of factual information that seldom need changing); journal subscriptions: general, specialized, and summary journals; a "personal collection" of material to support routine clinical and other usual activities (for example, a personal reprint collection or a specialized database of articles related to your clinical practice); a MEDLINE or other large database service for nonroutine topics that are often not covered by the sources from the first three categories; and an Internet connection.

TEXTBOOKS

Books were once the main repositories of reports of original research, but since the advent of journals they have usually included summaries of broad topics or tables of factual information or data. Often the information in books is "established" knowledge that is not subject to rapid change (for example, gross anatomy rather than drug regimens for prevention of progression of HIV infection or AIDS). Books are vital for students and for anyone who is interested in comprehensive summaries of areas of knowledge. Two examples of broad coverage of chapters in a text are congenital disorders of the biliary tract and pancreas, and managing psychiatric emergencies in primary care. Examples of facts that can come from a book are the gross anatomy of the elbow, the incubation period of chicken pox, normal developmental milestones for 3-, 4-, and 5-month old infants, and the prevalence of osteoarthritis in Norway.

Books are often 1 to 2 years out of date when published because of the time it takes to produce, print, and distribute them.

Another criticism is that the authors seldom provide enough data from studies or cite appropriate evidence sources to support their statements. Several publishers have developed new products or presentations of established products that overcome these two criticisms. In the medical field, *Scientific American Medicine*[20] and *UpToDate*[21] are two excellent examples of valuable evidence-based texts. *Scientific American Medicine* is a large, multichaptered book with many authors available in print, CD-ROM, and Internet-based text. It is updated regularly using mailed looseleaf pages for the print version, updated disks, and the Internet. In addition, authors are encouraged to link their statements to citations that provide the evidence to back them up.

UpToDate is an electronic text that has no print equivalent. It is a CD-ROM-based product for clinicians that presents its data in a "card" or question and answer format— synopses of information organized to answer specific clinical questions and provide recommendations for therapy. Almost 1500 editors and authors identify current advances in the literature and continuously update the material using literature searches and scanning of more than 130 clinical journals. Disk updates are provided quarterly. Text material is supplemented by MEDLINE citations, case presentations, slides, radiograms, electrocardiograms, and movies, any of which can be easily extracted for use in one's own presentations and teaching. Sildenafil (Viagra) was released on the U.S. market in mid-April, 1998 and by the summer *UpToDate* had comprehensive material supporting its use for sexual dysfunction in men. Many clinicians are coming to value this product. Similar "texts" will likely be developed in other fields, with further advances in provision of factual information. Clinicians need this text-based information daily, and choices should be a matter of personal preference. Care must be taken to ensure that the texts are appropriate, support routine work, and are kept current.

JOURNALS

Clinicians need journals to keep them up-to-date with professional news, governmental policy changes, and trends in research and practice, and to improve communication with other researchers, administrators, and peers. Haynes et al.[22,23] provide a broad description of the role of journal subscriptions, problems and challenges of journals, and how to choose titles. Although these papers are more than 10 years old, the basic ideas and premises are current, even with the advent of electronic journals and the Internet.

When you choose the journals to which you would like to subscribe, remember that almost all important advances in any health care discipline are published in the general medical journals: *New England Journal of Medicine, Lancet, JAMA,* and *BMJ.* Nurses, physiotherapists, occupational therapists, and members of allied health professions often do not consider that "their" major advances are published in these "big four" journals.

When it comes time to subscribe, new secondary publications are now available that provide abstracts and commentaries of published clinically applicable research. Articles are chosen based on the strict quality criteria that form the basis of this book. Current examples are *ACP Journal Club, Evidence-Based Medicine, Evidence-Based Cardiovascular Medicine, Evidence-Based Nursing, Evidence-Based Mental Health,* and *Evidence-Based Health Policy and Management.* Haynes describes in an editorial the rationale of starting the first one—*ACP Journal Club*—fast, accurate, yet short, presentation of the study, its results, and clinical applicability.[24] He states that the journal staff collect and present the articles most pertinent to the field of internal medicine that meet specific criteria, including clinical applicability and validity (methods sufficiently strong to support direct clinical application). Each article is abstracted in a structured form, and a commentary by an expert clinician is added that puts the study results in clinical perspective. Each article is allocated to one page in the evidence-based journal. Translations of the journals have been done, and total combined subscriptions are over 200,000, indicating that they are being used in practice. Also, several speciality journals, such as *American Journal of Sports Medicine,* and *Pediatrics,* devote sections to similar summaries of important new advances in their areas of health care.

A combination of general health care journals, such as one or more of the "big four," a journal or two from a clinician's discipline (for example, *Canadian Nurse* or *Canadian Medical Association Journal,* and, potentially, a summary journal probably provide sufficient journal coverage for most clinicians.

A PERSONAL COLLECTION

A personal collection of material to support everyday clinical practice is also important. Traditionally, this support has been provided by the development of a reprint collection or personal filing system. Again Haynes and colleague[25] describe how these collections can be designed and maintained. With the development and spread of fast, efficient database systems (for example, PubMed for MEDLINE) and the spread of fast, efficient home computers, these time-consuming reprint filing systems are becoming less common. While their importance fades other specialized collections of material are being developed to replace them. Sackett and Straus[26] describe two collections of summary documents they have developed in conjunction with medical and other students they have worked with in North America and the U. K. The *Red Book* and *CATs* (*Critically Appraised Topics*) are based on short written summaries of their clinical experience with internal medicine patients. They found that the *Red Book* successfully produced clinical answers for 39 of 39 care-based searches, and took an average of 10 seconds per search. *Critically Appraised Topics* was successfully searched 21 of 21 times, and took an average of 12 seconds per search.

Commercial products that provide a similar service of informing day-to-day clinical practice are now available. For example, *Best Evidence 3*[27] is a computer compilation of the material from *ACP Journal Club* (1991 to 1998) and from *Evidence-Based Medicine* (1995 to 1998). *Best Evidence* includes summary abstracts and commentaries from approximately 2200 original studies and systematic review articles published in over 150 important clinical journals. Each summer, material that is 5 years old is reviewed and updated or archived as needed. Each article meets stringent methodologic requirements, and has clinically important results. Sackett and Straus found that searching in *Best Evidence* took 26 seconds per search, considerably longer than for searching the *Red Book* or *CATs*; but it was still faster than a trip to the library or a MEDLINE search. Searching in *Best Evidence* is fast and easy because of its small size and its concentration of clinically relevant studies.

The *Cochrane Library* is another high-quality information product. Information about the Cochrane Collaboration and its role in collecting and producing systematic reviews is discussed in chapter 6, Secondary Publications—Systematic Review Articles. The *Library* is a CD-ROM and Internet product that contains evidence appropriate for making clinical decisions related to therapy, prevention, and quality improvement. It includes six separate sections and is updated quarterly. Three of the sections contain the full text of documents, and three are bibliographic collections (citations and abstracts of publications that are available elsewhere). The fourth quarterly update for 1998 of the *Library* includes 481 full-text systematic reviews, and a similar number of proposed and partially completed systematic reviews of important clinical topics related to issues across all disciplines of health care. This section of the *Cochrane Library* is probably the most important and clinically useful. It includes broad and narrow topics, such as: the effects of formal stroke units to reduce short- and long-term mortality; the best form of compression bandages to treat venous leg ulcers; how to improve our patients' adherence to their medications or appointment keeping; the effectiveness of St. John's wort for depression; and, the best topical agent for cord care in newborn infants. The second most useful section includes citations, often with abstracts, to 1820 systematic review articles produced by other research groups or individuals. This section of citations to other systematic review articles, called the *Database of Abstracts of Reviews of Effectiveness*, is updated regularly and is being expanded and constantly improved by staff at the University of York in the U. K. The third section is a clinical trials bibliographic database of more than 218,000 articles: randomized, controlled trials and controlled clinical trials as far back as the late nineteenth century. This section is produced and maintained by many persons using multiple comprehensive database searches and hand searching of important health care journals. The fourth section is a collection of citations to methodology articles; the fifth section has information for contacting individuals and groups within the Cochrane Collaboration; and the sixth section is the *Cochrane Handbook*, a working document for anyone interested in producing or understanding systematic reviews. The *Handbook* includes chapters on comprehensive searching accompanied by complex and effective searching strategies.

As described by Sackett and Straus,[26] clinicians need fast and efficient information support for their daily clinical encounters. Personal reprint filing systems have in the past provided this backup, but with the advent of new data transfer technology and an integration of better understanding of the information provision process with EBHC principles, we now have new personal and commercial information products. Two well-done examples are *Best Evidence 3* and the *Cochrane Library*.

LARGE BIBLIOGRAPHIC SEARCHING SYSTEMS (SUCH AS MEDLINE)

The products that provide extremely fast and effective support for everyday clinical encounters usually do not provide adequate coverage of topics rarely seen by a given clinician, or any clinician at all for that matter. Examples of this sort of information need would be a surgeon who is considering major surgery for an adult with a congenital malformation that in the past would have been fatal at birth (for example, CHARGE association), or new topics such as inflammation being associated with the development of atherosclerosis, the re-emergence of tuberculosis or diphtheria, and the public health consequences of the breakup of the U.S.S.R. The large bibliographic databases, such as MEDLINE, CINAHL, PsycINFO, and EMBASE/Excerpta Medica, were designed to provide broad coverage of all areas of health care, and therefore can provide this needed coverage of nonroutine or rare topics.

MEDLINE is the database produced by the National Library of Medicine in Bethesda, Maryland, U.S.A. Its paper equilavent is *Index Medicus*. It goes back to 1966, and includes more than nine million citations from over 4000 journals. It is designed to include citations to all health care literature, and is used heavily by physicians, nurses, other allied health care providers, researchers, students, patients, families, administrators, legal personnel, and journalists: almost anyone with an interest in health care. Many ways exist to access MEDLINE, and some of the more popular ones are PubMed *(http: //www.ncbi.nlm.nih.gov/PubMed/)*, Internet Grateful Med *(http://igm.nlm.nih.gov/)*, Ovid MEDLINE *(http://gateway.ovid.com/)*, and Knowledge Finder from Aries Systems Corportation *(http://www.kfinder.com/)*. Other MEDLINE access sites are available through Dr. Felix's Free MEDLINE pages *(http://www.beaker.iupui.edu/drfelix/, http://www.beaker.iupui.edu/drfelix/foreign.html*, and *http://www.docnet.org.uk/drfelix/)*.

CINAHL is a smaller database of material related to nursing and the other allied health disciplines. It is produced by a commercial company, CINAHL Information Systems and its paper equivalent has the same title. The database is smaller than MEDLINE, with over 300,000 records from 600 journals, books, and theses from 1982 on. Although smaller, it is a much "richer" database, with many enhancements of the traditional bibliographic information, including the full text of articles and other materials such as clinical practice guidelines, the bibliographies of many important articles, comments, book reviews, evaluations of multimedia and computer programs and systems, and patient education materials. More information, including access sites, can be found at *www.cinahl.com/*.

The PsycINFO database is produced by the American Psychological Association, and contains more than 1.5 million references to psychological literature from 1887 although its coverage is mainly from 1967 on. It includes more than the citations in *Psychological Abstracts* and the CD-ROM product is called PsycLIT. It is updated monthly, with approximately 5500 new references, and contains citations and abstracts to all types of publications of psychologically relevant material, including journal articles, dissertations, reports, English-language book chapters and books, and other scholarly documents. The database also includes literature from other disciplines related to psychology: education, business, medicine, nursing, law, and social work. More information is available at *http://www.apa.org/psycinfo/*.

EMBASE, the Excerpta Medica database, is a biomedical and pharmacologic database of medical and drug-related journal articles. Its paper equivalent are the *Excerpta Medica* indexes. Currently it has more than seven million citations, with 400,000 added annually (3800 journals). EMBASE's strengths are the inclusion of drug-related studies and European health care material, as well as extensive coverage of human medicine, research, allied health, alternative health, and health policy. More information is available at *http://www.elsevier.com/inca/publications/store/5/2/3/3/2/8/index.htt*. EMBASE and MEDLINE often have complimentary coverage of topics.

All of these databases are searched using similar techniques, although each has its own special features and specific searching techniques. Further, only MEDLINE is provided free on the Internet. Most people with a university or hospital affiliation, however, have access to most of these databases. Each database includes citations to journal articles and other, similar material. Searching can be done using author names and words or phrases in the title or abstract of the article. These words or phrases provided by the authors are often referred to as textwords, and are entered into the database just as they are printed in the journals. Each article is also indexed (given index terms, subject headings, or key words) using a standardized, controlled vocabulary developed by the database producers (for example bedsores are indexed as pressure sores in CINAHL, decubitus ulcers in MEDLINE, and decubitus in EMBASE—PsycINFO does not have a term for this idea or concept). Both textwords and index terms (subject headings) are used in effective searching, and specific words and terms to retrieve clinically relevant studies are listed in the tables of textwords and index terms for the databases in each of the major chapters. Textwords are especially useful for "new" terms or when you want to be comprehensive. Examples of "new" terms would be *secondhand smoke, Hurricane Mitch*, or *Kosovo*. Textwords can also be truncated to pick up multiple endings. *Random:* will retrieve *random, randomly, randomized,* and *randomised*. *Risk* will retrieve *risk, risks, risky*, and *risked*. Be careful, however, when you truncate. The term *salmon:* will, indeed, get *salmonella* and *salmonellae*, but it will also retrieve *salmon* the fish and *salmon sandwiches*. Index terms or subject headings are often most useful when the idea or concept is well defined in the literature: myocardial infarction, ACE inhibitors, and United States of America.

One effective feature of searching using index terms is the "explode" feature. When you search using a broad "umbrella" term such as *antibiotics, heart valves*, or *sports*, you must tell some MEDLINE searching systems that you want all the subsections of a broad term. For example, if you want all the sports terms in MEDLINE (i.e., *baseball, basketball, boxing* through to *rowing, skiing, skipping*, and *wrestling*) you must tell the searching program that you want to "explode" the term to get, or gather, all the terms together. In MEDLINE, the general term sports retrieves 1577 citations for 1995 to 1998; the term sports exploded has 6962 articles. Heart valves retrieves 341 articles; explode heart valves retrieves 4292 articles.

Textwords and index terms are "combined" using Boolean operators. The most often used operators are AND and OR. AND is used when you want to retrieve citations that have all the important concepts present. For example, in a search for information on the cost-effectiveness of warfarin and aspirin for patients with atrial fibrillation, a relevant citation would address all four ideas (*cost* AND *warfarin* AND *aspirin* AND *atrial fibrillation*). The ANDs make the retrievals smaller and more precise. If we wanted to be more precise for this search, we could AND in the requirement that data from a randomized trial were used (AND *randomized controlled trial*).

In contrast, when you use the OR operator you make your retrieval broader. If you were interested in using **any** of several nondrug therapies for treating migraine headache pain, you would AND migraine headache with any of the terms representing the therapies (*acupuncture* OR *exercise* OR *yoga* OR *relaxation* OR *stress reduction* OR *biofeedback* OR *humor*).

Some of the large databases also allow you to search using designations of what a citation "is." This is often referred to as a "publication type." For example, we can search MEDLINE for citations that are clinical trials (clinical trial [publication type]), and in CINAHL for citations that are research projects (research [publication type]). We use examples of these publication types in most of the tables of searching terms in all chapters. They are very effective for identifying for high-quality therapy studies and systematic review articles.

Because of the multitude of companies and institutions that provide searching programs for these databases, the above descriptions are generic in nature. Refer to the manuals and resource people at your institutions for full instructions on how to apply these techniques in the system or systems you have available. Many examples are also included in the CD-ROM at the back of this book.

THE INTERNET

The Internet is fast becoming a health care information source for clinicians and other health care professionals and for lay persons, patients, and their families and friends. The Internet offers myriad Websites, electronic mail lists, and online support groups. Mitchell et al.[28] addresses the need, and the desire of many patients and their families to obtain information on their disease or condition, by defining information therapy as, "the therapeutic provision of information to people for the amelioration of physical and mental health and well-being." This desire has roots in bibliotherapy, patient education, consumer health movements, patient's rights and the U.S. Freedom of Information Act. Identifying relevant information on the Internet may not be easy, but evaluating what you do find may be even more difficult. Some of the quality issues we describe in the following chapters may be used to evaluate Websites (for example, randomized controlled trials for therapy questions, and provision of search strategies and inclusion and exclusion criteria for systematic review articles).

Although some of the information on the Internet is similar to that in journal articles, much is different in that it is uncontrolled, often not peer reviewed, and may not include author names or affiliations. Getting started on the Internet looks complicated, but is not all that difficult. You need a fairly fast computer, a hookup to the Internet (a telephone line and modem or direct connection), software, and access through a commercial or institution Internet provider. The Internet provider can give you computer advice, and provide software, training, and ongoing help. Ask colleagues or the systems people where you work for recommendations and shop around.

As with all types of information it is important that you be able to assess the quality of the information you find before you decide whether to use it. This is even more important on the Internet where many of the quality enhancing aspects of journal publishing such as peer review, author listings, and funding sources and conflict of interest statements are not provided (i.e., anyone can set up an electronic journal and anyone can publish anything they want in it). To start to address the issue of evaluating quality on the Internet, Jadad and Gagliardi[29] wanted to identify rating instruments that had been used to evaluate health-related Internet sites. To collect these instruments they surveyed the Internet, completed multiple literature searches from six bibliographic databases, hand-searched several journals and collections of conference proceedings, and contacted experts and other interested parties using electronic discussion groups. They found 47 rating instruments, of which 14 provided the rating criteria. A fuller description of these 14 rating instruments is available on the Internet *(http://hiru.mcmaster.ca/ ebm/rating/table_3.htm)*.

Quality criteria for Internet sites can include any of:

- Attributes of authorship (individual or corporate authors);
- Disclosure of funding source or sources;
- Regular updating of material;
- Statements linked to supporting evidence, or at least the citation to supporting evidence;
- Endorsement by respected individuals or organizations.

Other attributes of sites that could reflect quality are high usage, personal endorsements by patients or family, and receipt of recognized awards. Common sense and your own experience are other quality assessment tools that should be applied whenever you use Web-based material. Just because something has been found on the Internet does not make it true. Many quality and retrieval issues wait to be addressed, but the Internet is here to stay for provision of information.

SUMMARY

Information retrieval is a skill. As with any skill, the most effective way of learning is to start in. Peers and librarians are good teachers and co-learners, and many classes and courses exist. We are all learners in this process because of the speed at which new knowledge accumulates, and the pace of new technology and services. A good adage to keep in mind is that those who are making mistakes are, likely, the only ones who are learning and changing.

CONTENT SEARCHING VERSUS METHODOLOGY SEARCHING

MEDLINE and other database searching is usually subject or content-based. Searches are done for drugs, diseases, syndromes, authors, and so on, with concepts put together in various Boolean combinations. These content-based searches do not differentiate among levels on the publication wedge—the idea paper, wet laboratory report, animal testing results and human studies that include the content will all be retrieved. Subject searching is appropriate for research needs (for example, retrieving everything on CD4$^+$ cell counts predicting mortality in patients with AIDS), but *not* for clinical needs (for example, several good papers on starting zidovudine combined with other drugs in patients with AIDS who have low CD4$^+$ cell counts). The material at the point of the wedge (clinical trials) is unique in the methods used to conduct the research. Computer searching can be harnessed to retrieve only citations of studies with a specific methodology. If we understand the basic methodologies of clinical research we can go beyond simple subject or content searching. We can use strategies to retrieve only the articles that are ready-for-application (EBHC): the ones at the narrowest point of the wedge, often referred to as clinical research.

CLINICAL RESEARCH

Robert and Suzanne Fletcher,[30] past coeditors of *Annals of Internal Medicine* and now at Harvard University, describe clinical research as follows:

> "Clinical research must provide sound data that clinicians can rely on in making decisions about patients. This kind of research should help to establish a body of knowledge that is useful in answering the following clinical questions: What medical condition does the patient have? How common is the condition? What are its causes? What is its prognosis? And how effective and risky is the treatment? Presumably, clinicians read original research published in medical journals to find answers to such questions."

To understand clinical research it is useful to study its history and stages, as we did for scientific communication.

History of Clinical Research

Clinical research has a long history;[31,32] the first recorded clinical trial is in the Bible, in Daniel 1:6 to 16. Daniel and his companions did not want to eat the rich food, that included meat and wine, common in the court of mighty King Nebuchadnezzar (the problem). They asked the prince of eunuchs to give them vegetables and water and not the palace food (the intervention). The chief eunuch reluctantly agreed, and after 10 days the king asked for Daniel and his friends to be brought in (the outcome assessment). The king found that none of the other young men in the palace were as healthy-looking as Daniel, Hananiah, Mishael, and Azariah, and kept them in his court for many years.

Grimes[33] assesses the strengths and weakness of this "trial" using modern standards, and contends that this Babylonian trial was good research with flaws common in studies today. Although his article is somewhat tongue-in-cheek, Grimes contends that the Daniel study has many strengths, including a contemporary control group (others in the court), blinded outcome assessment by the king, and the "striking brevity of the report." The weaknesses, according to Grimes, included a long lag time between execution of the study and publication, no randomization, and confounding of the study by divine intervention.

Scurvy

The first reported controlled therapy trial took place in the United Kingdom in 1747. Since the early 1600s, many people felt that citrus fruits might reduce the incidence of scurvy during long ocean voyages. Lind studied 12 sailors with scurvy, evaluating six potential treatments (Figure 1–2). Two sailors were given sea water, two were given vinegar, two were given lemons and limes, two were given elixir vitriol (copper sulfate), two were given a garlic and mustard mixture, and two were given cider. The two sailors who received the citrus fruits got better.[32] Although the results of this early trial were effective, low-cost, and easy to implement, the innovation was not adopted by the British Navy until 1795. The intervention was effective, however, and helped Britain gain dominance over the seas.

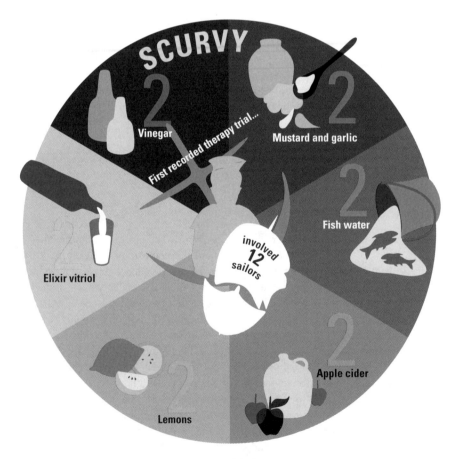

Figure 1–2 The first reported controlled therapy trial.

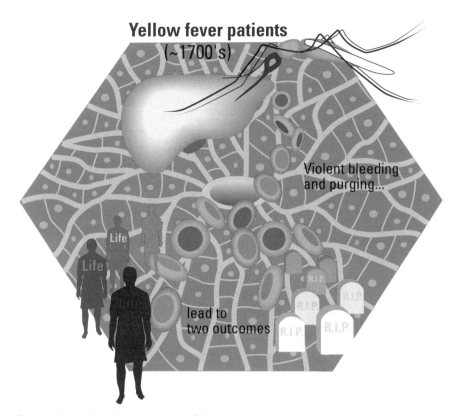

Figure 1–3 Another eighteenth century trial.

Yellow Fever

Another trial in the same century used *no* controls (Figure 1–3). The investigator treated patients with yellow fever with strong purging and bleeding. Many of his patients died, and the ones that did get better did so probably *despite* the therapy. On the basis of the results of this trial, yellow fever treatment using violent bleeding and purging was not changed for many years, and both mortality and morbidity remained high. If the investigator had used a control group, as Lind had done, the standard treatment for yellow fever might have been different.

Cold Vaccines

Methodologies have developed since the scurvy and yellow fever trials, and have matured in the past several decades. Both the United States and the United Kingdom contend that they were the developers of the randomized controlled trial. Cross-Atlantic research has been done to ascertain which country was the winner in the trials race. The U.S. contender for the first randomized controlled trial was one done and published by Diehl et al. in 1938. They studied cold vaccines in 498 university students at the University of Minnesota.[34] Half of the students received vaccinations and half received identical placebo injections. Both groups reported substantial reductions in the number of colds in the year after vaccination compared with the previous year, but the incidence rates for colds were similar in both groups both at baseline and at the end of the trial. The research program continued over many years and throughout many trials, but cold vaccinations were never shown to be effective and are not used now.

The results of the 1938 study were presented by Dr. Diehl at a conference, and the ensuing discussion was transcribed and published in *JAMA* as part of the paper. The discussion could have taken place today. The first person talks about the "strength of evidence" and many other discussants commented on control group and placebo effects. Historians cannot tell, however, if the trial was randomized, even after checking the original trial documents in the university archives and the historical collection of material at the U.S. National Library of Medicine. It was finally decided that the trial was not randomized. Even though the United States had the first entry 10 years before the U.K. entry, the race for the first randomized control led trial was won by Britain.

Streptomycin for Tuberculosis

The first truly randomized controlled trial was done in the United Kingdom and published by the *British Medical Journal* in 1948 (Figure 1–4). The British Medical Research Council's trial of streptomycin for tuberculosis[35] is considered a milestone in health care research. A major conference, entitled *50 Years of Clinical Trials*, was held in October 1998 to commemorate the fiftieth anniversary of its publication. Funding for the conference came from the British Medical Association, *BMJ* Publishing Group, and the U.K. Medical Research Council. Planners came from the United States, the United Kingdom, and Denmark. The themes of the conference reflect current thinking on health care research:

- Historical development of health care evaluation.
- International differences in approaches to health care evaluation.
- Interdisciplinary differences in evaluation.
- Politics of randomized controlled trials.
- Consumer participation in randomized controlled trials.
- Industry, government regulation, and clinical trials.
- Quality of randomized controlled trials.
- Statistical aspects of randomized controlled trials.
- The everyday business of running randomized controlled trials.
- Trials of historical and/or methodologic significance.
- How trials affect clinical practice.
- Trials and health policy: priorities and clinical trials.
- The future of health care evaluation.

Interestingly, the impetus for the 1948 streptomycin study did not come from the desire to advance scientific methodology, but because the medical staff had only half of the streptomycin needed for all patients with tuberculosis. The drug had been developed and tested during World War II, and after the war streptomycin testing moved from wound care to tuberculosis. The Medical Research Council staff felt that the fairest allocation method to decide who would receive the drug would be by chance alone, and therefore randomization to treatment groups was done (Each person had a 50% chance of receiving streptomycin or the placebo). Streptomycin was effective in curing tuberculosis, and soon many sanatoriums were closed throughout the United Kingdom, the Commonwealth, and the world. This trial became the recognized standard for health care researchers for many years, and embodies many of the techniques, policies, and procedures used in current health care research. It is also interesting to note that, in place of the abstract, a summary of research staff and meeting dates are given, and that at least one woman, Isabella Purdie, was part of the study team.

Smoking and Lung Cancer

The *British Medical Journal* also published another "first," this time in the area of etiology and causation. The question of cause-and-effect is an important one in health care, as are

---

BRITISH MEDICAL JOURNAL

LONDON SATURDAY OCTOBER 30 1948

STREPTOMYCIN TREATMENT OF PULMONARY TUBERCULOSIS
A MEDICAL RESEARCH COUNCIL INVESTIGATION

The following gives the short-term results of a controlled investigation into the effects of streptomycin on one type of pulmonary tuberculosis. The inquiry was planned and directed by the Streptomycin in Tuberculosis Trials Committee, composed of the following members: Dr. Geoffrey Marshall (chairman), Professor J. W. S. Blacklock, Professor C. Cameron, Professor N. B. Capon, Dr. R. Cruickshank, Professor J. H. Gaddum, Dr. F. R. G. Heaf, Professor A. Bradford Hill. Dr. L. E. Houghton, Dr. J. Clifford Hoyle, Professor H. Raistrick, Dr. J. G. Scadding, Professor W. H. Tytler, Professor G. S. Wilson, and Dr. P. D'Arcy Hart (secretary). The centres at which the work was carried out and the specialists in charge of patients and pathological work were as follows:

Brompton Hospital, London.—Clinician: Dr. J. W. Crofton, Streptomycin Registrar (working under the direction of the honorary staff of Brompton Hospital): Pathologists: Dr. J. W. Clegg, Dr. D. A. Mitchison.
 Colindale Hospital (L.C.C.), London.—Clinicians: Dr. J. V. Hurford, Dr. B. J. Douglas Smith, Dr. W. E. Snell : Pathologists (Central Public Health Laboratory): Dr. G. B. Forbes, Dr. H. D. Holt.
 Harefield Hospital (M.C.C.), Harefield, Middlesex.— Clinicians: Dr. R. H. Brent, Dr. L. E. Houghton; Pathologist: Dr. E. Nassau.

Bangour Hospital, Bangour, West Lothian.—Clinician: Dr. I. D. Ross ; Pathologist: Dr. Isabella Purdie.
 Killingbeck Hospital and Sanatorium, Leeds.—Clinicians: Dr. W. Santon Gilmour, Dr. A. M. Reevie ; Pathologist: Professor J. W. McLeod.
 Northern Hospital (L.C.C.), Winchmore Hill, London.—Clinicians: Dr. F. A. Nash, Dr. R. Shoulman ; Pathologists: Dr. J. M. Alston, Dr. A. Mohun.
 Sully Hospital, Sully, Glam.—Clinicians: Dr. D. M. E. Thomas, Dr. L. R. West ; Pathologist: Professor W. H. Tytler.

The clinicians of the centres met periodically as a working subcommittee under the chairmanship of Dr. Geoffrey Marshall ; so also did the pathologists under the chairmanship of Dr. R. Cruickshank. Dr. P. D'Arcy Daniels, of the Council's scientific staff, was responsible for the clinical co-ordination of the trials, and he also prepared the report for the Committee, with assistance from Dr. D. A. Mitchison on the analysis of laboratory results. For the purpose of final analysis the radiological findings were assessed by a panel composed of Dr. L. G. Blair, Dr. Peter Kerley, and Dr. Geoffrey S. Todd.

Figure 1–4 Publication of the first truly randomized control trial. This page was first published in the BMJ (Medical Research Council Investigation: Streptomycin treatment of tuberculosis. Br Med J 1948;2:769–82) and is used with permission of the BMJ.

REPORT ON CERTAIN ENTERIC FEVER INOCULATION STATISTICS.

PROVIDED BY LIEUTENANT-COLONEL R. J. S. SIMPSON, C.M.G., R.A.M.C.

By KARL PEARSON, F.R.S.,
Professor of Applied Mathematics, University College, London.

THE statistics in question were of two classes : (A) Incidence (B) Mortality Statistics. Under each of these headings the data belonged to two groups : (i) Indian experience; (ii) South African War experience. These two experiences were of a somewhat different character. That for India covered apparently the European army, of whatever branch and wherever distributed; that for South Africa was given partly by locality, partly by column, and partly by special hospital. Thus the Indian and South African experiences seem hardly comparable. Many of the groups in the South African experience are far too small to allow of any definite opinion being formed at all, having regard to the size of the probable error involved. Accordingly, it was needful to group them into larger series. Even thus the material appears to be so heterogeneous, and the results so irregular, that it must be doubtful how much weight is to be attributed to the different results.

The following groups were made on the basis of Lieutenant-Colonel Simpson's table (see Appendix A).

A. Incidence.

South Africa :
    I. Hospital Staffs. See Appendix B, Table (1).
    II. Garrison of Ladysmith. See Appendix B, Table (2).
    III. Methuen's Column. See Appendix B, Table (3).
    IV. Group of three special Regiments : 7th Hussars, C.I.V.'s, and 5th Battalion Manchesters. See Appendix B, Table (4).
India :
    V. Army in India. Here I have taken only the data for years 1900 and 1901, as I am told that the statistics for 1899 are not fully comparable with those for the two later years. See Appendix B, Table (5).

B. Mortality.

South Africa :
    I. Hospital Staffs. See Appendix B, Table (6).
    II. Garrison of Ladysmith.* See Appendix B, Table (7).
    III. Special Regiments. See Appendix B, Table (8).
    IV. Group of special Hospitals, South Africa. See Appendix B, Table (9).
    V. Various military Hospitals. See Appendix B, Table (10).
India :
    VI. Army in India, 1900-1. See Appendix B, Table (11).

* No mortality experience was given in the case of Methuen's column.

Figure 1–5 One of the first studies to combine data from various trials. This page was first published in the BMJ (Pearson K. Report on certain enteric fever inoculation statistics. Br Med J 1904;3:1243–6) and is used with permission of the BMJ.

the questions of how to diagnose and treat diseases and conditions and understand their progression. One of the first well-done causation studies, published in 1950, formally assessed why the rates of lung cancer seemed to be increasing in England and Wales after World War II. Deaths from lung cancer had gone from 612 in 1922 to 9287 in 1947. Doll and Hill[36] studied general atmospheric pollution from the exhaust fumes of cars, the surface dust of tarred roads, and smoke and residue from industrial plants and coal fires, plus the smoking of tobacco. They developed a new study design, called a case-control study. "Cases," those with lung cancer, were matched and compared with "controls," those without it. The rates of exposure to the pollution and various kinds of smoke were compared in cases and controls, and conclusions drawn. By the end of their case-control study, Doll and Hill felt confident that tobacco smoking, and not tarred roads or industrial pollution, was associated with the large increase in lung cancer deaths.

Both Doll and Hill were knighted for their innovative and groundbreaking work in the area of tobacco smoke pollution and also for their work at improving and perfecting health care research methods. Both continued to produce high quality health care research and train many generations of British researchers. Although Sir Bradford Hill has died, Richard Doll is still associated with the Radcliffe Infirmary of Oxford University, United Kingdom and continues to lecture, teach and conduct research.

Systematic Review Articles

One of the first studies to combine data from various trials—the forerunner of modern meta-analyses—is also from the *British Medical Journal*. Karl Pearson[37] published a report in 1904 that combined enteric fever statistics from several sources (Figure 1–5). He combined data from four reports of incidence data from the British Army in South Africa and one from the British Army in India. For mortality, he added another set of data from South Africa. It is interesting that even though his article was short and included several tables and did not have an abstract, introduction, or references, it included a discussion of the ideas of homogeneity of the data (are the data similar enough to combine in one analysis?) and of weighting the values in the data sets by study size. Both concepts are vitally important to modern-day meta-analysts, and they are discussed in the first paragraph of the study. Karl Pearson was a well known statistician at the turn of the century, and not a health care professional. He developed the Pearson coefficient that is heavily used today, along with many other important statistical concepts and methodologies, although he is not recognized as foundational in the development of systematic review articles.

U.S. Randomized Controlled Trial

One of the first large, multicenter, truly randomized controlled trials done in the United States was published in 1956 (Figure 1–6). It studied the optimal usage and dose of oxygen in small and premature babies.[38] Oxygen use and special care nurseries were saving premature infants' lives. In practice, because of the effectiveness of the oxygen, nurses and physicians were using increasing concentrations of oxygen in their desire to save

OPHTHALMOLOGY

Retrolental Fibroplasia

Cooperative Study of Retrolental Fibroplasia and the Use of Oxygen

V. EVERETT KINSEY, Ph.D.

Detroit

With the Assistance of June Twomey Jacobus, B.A., Detroit,
and F. M. Hemphill, Ph.D., Ann Arbor

Table of Contents

Received for publication July 27, 1956.

From the Kresge Eye Institute (Dr. Kinsey and Mrs. Jacobus) and the Department of Public Health Statistics, School of Public Health, University of Michigan (Dr. Hemphill).

The Cooperative Study of Retrolental Fibroplasia was supported in part by a grant from the National Institute for Neurological Diseases and Blindness of the U. S. Public Health Service, Bethesda, Md.; the National Foundation for Eye Research, Boston, and the National Society for the Prevention of Blindness, New York.

The Coordination Committee was composed of the following members: V. Everett Kinsey, Chairman, Kresge Eye Institute; Richard L. Day, State University of New York College of

(Footnotes continued on next page)

Figure 1–6 The first U.S. randomized controlled trial. Published with the permission of the American Medical Association, copyright 1956. (Kinsey VE. Retrolental fibroplasia. AMA Archives of Ophthalmology 1956;56:481–543).

even more premature babies. The babies were alive, but in a 5-year period in the late 1940s and early 1950s more than 10,000 U.S. babies had lost their sight. No one seemed to know why. Even the *Saturday Evening Post* tried to solve the mystery by commissioning and publishing a large investigative report. Kinsey et al. completed and published a scientifically sound dose-finding study, and established the best dose of oxygen to balance the benefits and harms of the therapy. Oxygen is now used as needed, and not routinely, and many fewer cases of blindness occur.

This study report, published in the *AMA Archives of Ophthalmology,* includes a table of contents for the 63-page article. Although this table of contents looks strange by today's standards, this is exactly the format used in electronic publishing of journal articles. One could argue, albeit with tongue in cheek, that the American Medical Association was getting ready for electronic publishing in 1956.

Summary of Current Clinical Research

Health care research has continued to evolve in the past 40–50 years and each category of research (especially therapy, diagnosis, etiology and causation, natural history and prognosis, economics, systematic reviews, and clinical practice guidelines) has developed its own unique set of research methods and techniques.

Two features, however, that all applied clinical research studies have in common are that they are comparative, and they are preplanned. The first, and probably most important, aspect is that they are comparative. Without valid and reliable comparisons between two or more groups, health care would be driven by opinions and current procedures rather than by true scientific advances. Remember back several pages to our example of yellow fever and the bleeding and purging. Examples of these comparisons for a therapy trial will be a comparison of persons taking one drug with persons taking another drug or placebo (for example, aspirin versus warfarin for stroke prevention in persons with atrial fibrillation). Treatment group (also called intervention or study group) participants are those who receive the active, new, or untested therapy. Control participants form the other comparison group(s). Control patients usually get standard treatment (or no treatment) instead of the experimental therapy.

A diagnosis study will compare the results of two or more diagnostic tests in persons with and without the disease in question (for example, thallium scanning versus cardiac enzyme measurements to assess whether patients who come to the emergency department with chest pain are actually having a myocardial infarction). An etiology and causation study compares persons exposed to some agent thought to cause a disease and those not exposed (for example, very elderly persons, some with and some without high levels of cholesterol, who are then compared to ascertain if high cholesterol levels are associated with longer survival for persons over the age of 85: they seem to be). For prognosis and natural history studies, the comparative feature is present, but less evident. The comparison is best addressed by the example of a woman who has just been told that she has multiple sclerosis. She wants to know if this disease will affect her life style or survival compared with what she could have expected if she did not have it. Economic analyses compare costs of implementing a new procedure with costs if the procedure had not been implemented.

Careful, comprehensive planning goes into research studies before they start. Initially, a research question is posed that takes into account the patient's disease or condition, procedure, duration, outcomes and so on. From this question, protocols are developed that include very specific details describing all aspects of the study. For example, all drug studies include dosages, administration routes, and timing (for example, 20 mg per day, four times daily, 1 hour before meals). They also include details for dealing with adverse reactions to the drugs, patient inclusion and exclusion criteria, how to encourage and measure patient compliance, how to deal with dropouts, what measures to use for evaluation, procedures for recruitment and follow-up of all patients, and processes and timing for all final evaluations of all patients. Diagnosis studies list in exact detail all procedures for the tests that are being studied (for example, how to ask and score the four questions used in the CAGE questionnaire to identify problem drinking: have you ever tried to *Cut* down on your drinking, has anyone ever been *Angry* at your drinking, have you ever felt *Guilty* about your drinking, and have you ever needed an *Eye-opener*?). Causation studies define exposures (for example, cigarette pack years). Prognosis studies define exact disease characteristics (for example, first episode of optic neuritis of more than 1 week duration in one or both eyes) and the outcomes (for example, multiple sclerosis based on MRI of lesions on the brain within 5 to 10 years of optic neuritis).

Here the similarities among the types of research studies end. Each of the following chapters will discuss a specific type of research and what distinguishes it beyond the shared characteristics of being comparative and preplanned.

REFERENCES

1. Oxman AD, Sackett DL, Guyatt GH, and the Evidence-Based Medicine Working Group. Users guides to the medical literature. JAMA 1993;270:2093–7.
2. Sackett DL, Haynes RB, Guyatt GH, Tugwell P. Clinical epidemiology: a basic science for clinical medicine. 2nd ed. Boston: Little, Brown; 1991.
3. Sackett DL, Rosenberg WMC, Gray MJA, et al. Evidence-based medicine: what it is and what is isn't. BMJ 1996;312:71–2.
4. Evidence-based medicine in its place [editorial]. Lancet 1995;346:785.
5. Feinstein AR, Horwitz RI. Problems in the "evidence" of "evidence-based medicine." Am J Med 1997;103:529–35.
6. De Solla Price D. The development and structure of the biomedical literature. In: Warren K, editor. Coping with the biomedical literature: a primer for the scientist and clinician. New York: Praeger; 1981. p. 3–16.
7. Southgate T. The cover. JAMA 1998;280:1552.
8. De Solla Price D. Communication in science: the ends—philosophy and forecast. In: De Reuck A, editor. Communication in science: documentation and automation. London: Churchill; 1967. p. 189–213.
9. Rennie J. Civilizing the Internet [editorial]. Sci Am 1997;276:6.
10. Britton TC. Increased writing activity in neurological disease. Lancet 1997:349:372–3.
11. Lantner RR, Ros SP. Blue jeans thighs. Pediatrics 1991;88:417.
12. Morgan WK. Zamboni disease. Arch Intern Med 1997;157:135.

13. Fain O, Mathieu E, Thomas F. Scurvy in patients with cancer. Lancet 1998;316:1661–2.
14. Galimand M, Guiyoule A, Gerbaud G, et al. Multidrug resistance in *Yersina pestis* mediated by a transferable plasmid. N Engl J Med 1997;337:667–8.
15. Muhlestein JB, Anerson JL, Hammond EH, et al. Infection with *Chlamydia pneumoniae* accelerated the development of atherosclerosis and treatment with azithromycin prevents it in an animal model. Circulation 1998;97:633–6.
16. Marcurad SP, Albernaz L, Khazaine PG. Omeprazole therapy causes malabsorption of cyanocobalamin (Vitamin B_{12}). Ann Intern Med 1994;120:211–5.
17. Schumacher B, Pecher P, von Specht BU, Stegmann T. Induction of neoangiogenesis in ischemic myocardium by human growth factors: first clinical results of a new treatment of coronary heart disease. Circulation 1998;97:645–50.
18. CLASP: a randomised trial of low-dose aspirin for the prevention and treatment of pre-eclampsia among 9364 pregnant women. Lancet 1994;343:619–29.
19. Matson E. Speed kills (the competition). Fast Company 1996 Aug/Sep(3):84–91.
20. Dale DC, Federman DD [editors]. Scientific American medicine. Scientific American: New York: 1999. Telephone 800-545-0554.
21. UpToDate Contact information: telephone 781-237-4788; fax: 781-239-0391; Web: www.uptodateinc.com.
22. Haynes RB, McKibbon KA, Fitzgerald D, et al. How to keep up with the medical literature. II. Deciding which journals to read regularly. Ann Intern Med 1986;105:309–12.
23. Haynes RB, McKibbon KA, Fitzgerald D, et al. How to keep up with the medical literature. Part III. Expanding the volume of literature you read regularly. Ann Intern Med 1986;105:474–8.
24. Haynes RB. The origins and aspirations of *ACP Journal Club* [editorial]. ACP J Club 1991 Jan–Feb; 114:A18–9.
25. Haynes RB, McKibbon KA, Fitzgerald D, et al. How to keep up with the medical literature. Part VI. How to store and retrieve articles worth keeping. Ann Intern Med 1986;105:978–84.
26. Sackett DL, Straus SE, for the Firm A of the Nuffield Department of Medicine. Finding and applying evidence during clinical rounds. The "Evidence Cart." JAMA 1998;280:1336–8.
27. Best Evidence 3 Telephone contact information: U.S.A. 800-523-1546; Canada 613-731-8610; United Kingdom 011-44-171-387-4499.
28. Mitchell DJ. Toward a definition of information therapy. Proc Annu Symp Comput Appl Med Care. 1994;71–5.
29. Jadad AR, Gagliardi A. Rating health information on the Internet. JAMA 1998;279:611–4.
30. Fletcher RH, Fletcher SW. Clinical research in general medical journals: a 30 year perspective. N Engl J Med 1979;301:180–3.
31. Spitzer WE, Feinstein AR, Sackett DL. What is a health care trial? JAMA 1967;233:161–3.
32. Jenkins J, Hubbard S. History of clinical trials. Semin Oncol Nursing 1991;7:228–34.
33. Grimes DA. Clinical research in ancient Babylon: methodologic insights from the Book of Daniel. Obstet Gynecol 1995;86:1031–4.
34. Diehl HS, Baker AB, Cowan AD. Cold vaccines: an evaluation based on a control study. JAMA 1938;111:1168–73.
35. Medical Research Council Investigation: Streptomycin treatment of tuberculosis. Br Med J 1948;2:769–82.
36. Doll R, Hill AB. Smoking and carcinoma of the lung: preliminary report. Br Med J 1950;2:740–8.
37. Pearson K. Report on certain enteric fever inoculation statistics. Br Med J 1904;3:1243–6.
38. Kinsey VE. Retrolental fibroplasia. Comparative study of retrolental fibroplasia and the use of oxygen. AMA Arch Ophthalmol 1956;56:481–543.

Therapy, Prevention and Control, and Quality Improvement

CLINICAL EXAMPLE OF MUSIC AND BRONCHOSCOPY

Research methodology is better understood with examples than by discussion of theory alone. In the study by Dubois et al.,[1] they wanted to understand and decrease the discomfort associated with bronchoscopy without increasing the risk of adverse effects. They wondered if letting the patients listen to music during the procedure would help them feel more comfortable. The project was planned and funding found to study 52 patients. Patients with an odd chart number were asked if they wanted to listen to music during the bronchoscopy. These patients formed the study or intervention group. Patients with even chart numbers were not given the option (the control group). Of the 24 people who were asked if they wanted music, 21 agreed to listen to Yanni's *Reflections of Passion*. The patients in the study group listened to the music using headphones during the bronchoscopy. Twenty-eight people formed the control group, and did not listen to music. Afterwards, all patients in both groups completed a questionnaire that used visual analog scales to report their levels of discomfort (put a mark on the scale to show how uncomfortable you felt). The comparison of music with no music allowed the researchers to ascertain if the music reduced discomfort during the procedure. Study outcomes were physiological responses, patient-reported discomfort, physician and technician perceptions of patient discomfort, and medication use.

Several interesting things were seen. First, three patients who were asked to be part of the music group did not take part in the study. This means that the follow-up of the study was 49/52, or 94%. Second, overall the patients in the music group found the bronchoscopy less uncomfortable (score 2.5 on the visual analog scale) than patients in the no-music group (score 3.5) ($P = .02$). "P" value means the probability of getting a different answer if we repeated the trial. For a p-value of .02 we would get the same answer (music was better) 98 times out of 100 repeats of the trial. Patients in the music group also had better cough scores ($P = .03$). Third, the physicians' and technicians' assessments of the discomfort of the patients bore little resemblance to what the patients reported. This difference between the assessment by the physicians and technicians and the patients' points out some of the problems with assessments and measurements of outcomes of studies. **Surrogate**, or indirect, measures of an outcome are not nearly as accurate or reliable as measurement of direct outcomes: the patients knew their personal discomfort far better than the health professionals who were watching the procedure.

HOW A THERAPY TRIAL IS DONE

A rigorous or well-done therapy trial starts with a group of persons, all of whom have the disease or condition that is to be studied. Two or more interventions or treatments are compared in the study population. To make this comparison as true and replicable as possible, patients are studied in two or more groups that are as equivalent as possible. Patients in each group take their allotted therapy (drug, surgery, music, placebo, and so on). After a specified period, researchers measure all outcomes in all participants and compare the groups. For a true comparison, these study groups must be as similar as possible in all respects *except for the treatment.*

The study design, or methodology, used for evaluating therapeutic, quality improvement, or prevention interventions is called a **randomized controlled trial** or a **controlled clinical trial.** Examples of prevention studies are the music study above, or training workshops combined with follow-up sessions at the start of each high school semester, given to teenaged boys and girls to reduce the rates of pregnancy and sexually transmitted diseases in the following semesters. An example of a therapy trial is the assessment of amoxicillin to cure otitis media. An example of a quality improvement trial is adding routine notes to the charts of ambulatory patients reminding clinicians of the need for women to be screened for breast cancer; another is implementing case managers in hospital wards to improve the care process as well as patient outcomes of increased satisfaction, shorter hospital stays, and lower infection rates after surgery.

RANDOMIZATION

To be sure that the groups are as similar as possible, patients are put into each study group using an allocation method that is unbiased (no personal preference on anyone's part is allowed). Random allocation is the best way to do this. Researchers use random number tables, coin tosses, or other, similar methods and set up allocation sequences for patients. This can be done before the study starts or done during the study itself. When a patient agrees to be part of the study and is ready to enter it, they get the *next* allocation, often in a sealed envelope or via a telephone call to the study office. Allocation by birth date, patient chart number, or day of week seen in the clinic is not random. These methods are, however, better than coin tosses or clinician or patient preference to ensure comparability of groups, as long as the allocation procedure is strictly adhered to; often however, it is not.

Randomization can be done with "parts" of people (for example half of head washed with shampoo A and half with shampoo B to assess softness or the ability to kill head lice, or arms randomly allocated to intravenous insertion of a catheter using the standard landmark guidance procedure or ultrasonography). Most often persons are allocated, but towns, wards, schools, hospitals, bus stops, and so on have been allocated. The research question often dictates the unit randomized.

Groups do not need to be the same size. Often the sizes are similar, but randomization does not guarantee exactly equal numbers. Indeed, some studies purposely involve unequal numbers. For example, Maizel et al.[2] studied intranasal lidocaine compared with placebo for migraine pain relief. Twice as many people (58:28) were allocated to receive the intranasal lidocaine as were allocated to receive placebo (intranasal saline solution). These unequal groups were formed because of the ethics and common sense issues of withholding medication from persons with migraine headache pain. The analysis at the end of the study can factor and adjust for the difference in group size.

BLINDING

In addition to the random allocation in therapy trials, patients, health care workers, and the study personnel should not know, if feasible, the group to which the patient is assigned. This is called blinding or masking and it avoids what is commonly called measurement bias. Human nature being what it is, patient *and* health care worker expectations are strong, and often unconsciously influence reporting of outcomes. Quite often, with the best of intentions, people report as truth what they think should be happening or what they expect others to think should be happening. To minimize these biased perceptions, neither the health care worker nor the patient should know which treatment a patient is receiving.

For example, an early vitamin C study was funded by the U.S. National Institutes of Health and the results were published in 1975.[3] This trial was to definitively prove what researchers had reported since 1938: that vitamin C was the wonder drug for the common cold. People were randomly given either vitamin C in capsules or powdered sucrose in similar capsules, and instructed to take them on the same, fixed schedule. They were to report all colds and related symptoms. Some study participants, knowing the taste difference between the vitamin C and sugar, opened the capsules and tasted them. (This is known as **code breaking**.) When people reported their outcomes—cold symptoms—they told the researchers that they had "broken the code." Knowing that some persons had discovered which group they were in, the researchers analyzed the data to compare rates of cold symptoms in the persons who knew what they were taking and in the persons who did not know—called a **subgroup analysis**. The rates of colds and symptoms did not differ in these two subgroups, indicating that the code breaking had not affected the results. Controversy continues however, around the results of the study and around questions of proper data analysis, assessment of other biases, code breaking, and trial methods, and researchers are still not confident they have completely evaluated whether vitamin C prevents or reduces the burden of the common cold.

Proper blinding takes much planning, preparation, and creativity. In one study comparing two drug treatments for lowering cholesterol, one drug needed to be taken once a day at bedtime. The other drug was taken three times a day at meals. Each person in the trial took four pills a day: one with each meal, and one at bedtime. Some were placebos and some were "real" medicine. Texture, taste, color, and other features were closely matched for placebo and active medicine. Some studies have gone to extremes to incorporate blinding. One surgery trial many years ago randomized patients to surgery or no-surgery after the patients had gone to the operating room, been prepped and anesthetized, and the operation started. When the patients were ready for the surgery to start, the surgeon received notification of the random allocation. Half the patients had surgery and the other half did not. For the people not randomized to the surgery group, the surgery was terminated and they were returned to their rooms to be given their drug treatment. Although creative, this type of blinding could not be done today because of ethical concerns and the growing awareness of patients' rights and obligations to full disclosure of information.

Single-, Double-, and Triple-Blinding

Three groups of persons are usually involved in health care studies: patients; their health care providers; and the study personnel. **Single blinding** usually refers to *either* the patient *or* the health professional not knowing the study allocation. **Double-blinding** usually refers to the health professional *and* the patient not knowing which medicine or study intervention the patient is receiving. **Triple-blinding** implies that the health professionals, the patient, *and* the study personnel, including the data management staff, do not know which treatment is active therapy and which is placebo or standard therapy until final data analysis is complete. Triple-blinding is very important for trials sponsored by drug companies. The companies are often criticized for putting their profits above reporting of negative trials of their products, and this full-scale triple-blinding helps all users of health care research to have confidence in final published results. Double-blinding is the most common form of blinding reported.

Blinding Not Always Possible

In some cases, it is not possible to blind a study because of logistical or ethical problems. For example, heart surgeons undertook surgery on both warm and cooled hearts in an unblinded study in Toronto.[4] Historically, surgeons thought chilled hearts needed less oxygen, and therefore suffered less tissue damage during operations than hearts that were kept at body temperature. Researchers disputed this, and a randomized controlled trial was done to determine whether this assumption was true. Because it was not possible to blind the surgeons to the temperature of the hearts they operated on, the researchers did not even try. Instead, they put their energies into making sure the outcomes measured (death, morbidity, time off work, and so on) were assessed in as unbiased a way as possible. To do this, neither the patients nor the persons who assessed the outcomes knew the procedure each patient received, and the surgeons were not involved in assessing any of the study outcomes related to the patients.

   Another example where blinding could not take place is a study of premature babies. Newborn babies, especially premature ones, do not regulate their internal temperatures well, and it is important for their bodies to be at a constant, normal temperature. A randomized controlled trial was undertaken in which babies were assigned to either higher thermostat settings on their isolets, or to wearing hats, on the assumption that most body heat is lost through one's head. During the interim and final assessments of the infants the babies were not wearing hats. They were also assessed by a study staff member who had no knowledge of each infant's hat status. The higher thermostat settings did more harm than good, and babies in most neonatal intensive care units now wear hats.[5]

Ophthalmologists and "Masked" Studies

Blinding also goes by other names. For example, ophthalmologists who deal with patients with vision problems prefer the term **masked**. Gwon et al. studied topical ofloxacin compared with gentamicin for treatment of internal ocular infection[6] and reported the blinding of their study using the term "masked." **Sham, dummy**, and **double dummy** are other terms that refer to placebos and blinding. They are used more often in European studies than in studies done in North America.

FOLLOW-UP

Participant follow-up is also very important in understanding, evaluating, and applying randomized controlled trial results. Most methodologists insist that at least 80% of all participants who were randomized at the start of the study are analyzed at the end of the study for the results to be valid or "true." This means accounting for all participants who withdrew from the treatments (keeping this number to a minimum), dropped out, or were otherwise lost. If more than 20% of the participants were lost because they became much better, or much worse, with specific treatments, the study's results might not be generalizable. (**Generalizability** is the degree to which the results can be taken from a specific research study and applied to other groups of persons—steps three and four in the five-step EBHC process.)

Attaining good follow-up can be easy or hard, depending on the study. An example of easy follow-up is a short-term study designed to assess the relative benefits of standard-dose intravenous pain relief with a patient-controlled arrangement using a pump injection system within the first 24 hours of cardiac surgery. Such a study would easily have a 100% follow-up rate. Follow-up is much more difficult when the study lasts longer, the patients are more mobile, and few incentives exist to keep patients interested. Examples of difficult follow-up would be a program to cure and prevent the spread of tuberculosis in homeless persons, and methadone and counseling studies over a period of years in persons with substance abuse problems.

UNDERSTANDING THERAPY STATISTICS

In addition to understanding how a therapy trial is done, and how it is indexed and reported in an abstract, anyone who is interested in health care or EBHC needs to know the common conventions authors use to report study outcomes. The following is a simple nonclinical example. Assume that the health care budget cuts are too difficult and frustrating, and you have decided that, instead of your present job, you want to start a cream cheese factory and produce a good-tasting, low-fat product. Your product tastes wonderful, and production costs seem to suggest your endeavors will be cost-effective. Marketing is your next step in getting the cheese on the grocery shelves. You tentatively call it "Lite-Bites." If the regular-fat cream cheese has a 40% butterfat content, and your low-fat Lite-Bites has a 20% butterfat content, how are you going to describe and advertise your product? You can describe the fat issues in the following ways:

- Your cream cheese has 20% less than theirs; or
- Theirs has 20% more butterfat than yours.

These two statistics represent an *absolute* difference (for example, from 40 to 20% is a 20% reduction, or from 20 to 40% is a 20% increase in butterfat).

We can also say that the difference is that:

- Yours has a 50% reduction in fat levels compared with theirs; or
- Theirs has a 100% increase in fat levels compared with yours.

These two statistics represent a *relative* difference. For example, starting at 40% and going to 20% cuts the fat in half—a 50% reduction, and going from 20 to 40% doubles the fat—a 100% increase. Both the two absolute differences (20%) and the two relative differences (50% and 100%) are correct representations of the differences in fat levels between the two brands of cream cheese.

Clinicians have many ways of describing the results of clinical trials: even more than the absolute and relative differences seen in the cream cheese example. Frick et al.[7] studied patients who had high levels of cholesterol. They wanted to lower the cholesterol levels and prevent myocardial infarction using the drug gemfibrozil. After 5 years they found that, in patients who had received placebo, 3.9% of the persons had had a myocardial infarction. For patients who had received gemfibrozil, the rate of myocardial infarction was 2.3%. The differences between, and the clinical implications of the 3.9% and 2.3% can be represented by any of the following seven statistics (The name of the statistic is in parentheses after the statistic itself):

- 1.6% fewer patients had myocardial infarctions (**absolute risk reduction**).
- 41% reduction in the rate of myocardial infarction (**relative risk reduction**).
- One would need to treat 71 patients for 5 years to prevent one additional patient from having a myocardial infarction (**number needed to treat**).
- 389,000 pills would have to be taken to prevent one additional patient from having a myocardial infarction (**number of pills needed to be taken**).
- Each patient treated increased their time with no myocardial infarction, on average by 15 weeks (**disease-free survival**).
- Each life-year saved cost U.S. $47,523 (**life-year cost savings**).
- Gemfibrozil is better than placebo ($P < .01$) (*P*-value comparison).

Hux and Naylor[8] gave 100 patients most of the above numbers and asked them to choose if they would take the study drug based on their perceptions of the accompanying numbers. Their responses are summarized below.

- The **absolute risk reduction** is 1.6% fewer deaths—the arithmetic difference between 3.9% and 2.3%. It is the simplest statistic. This is calculated as the difference in rates (3.9% − 2.3% = 1.6%). Forty-two percent of the participants in the survey by Hux and Naylor would choose to take gemfibrozil if they were give the absolute risk reduction numbers. This conceptually is identical to the 20% differences in the cream cheese example.
- The **relative risk reduction** is a 41% reduction—conceptually identical to the 50% and 100% calculated in the cream cheese example. This is calculated as the difference (1.6%) divided by the rate in the placebo group 1.6/3.9 = 41%. Even though this number is derived from the same data, 88% of the Hux and Naylor participants would choose to take gemfibrozil when given this relative risk reduction statistic.
- The **number (of persons) needed-to-treat** (NNT) is 71 to prevent one additional myocardial infarction at 5 years. Another way of putting this is that for every 71 patients who received gemfibrozil for 5 years, one additional myocardial infarction would be prevented. The NNT number is calculated by the formula

$$\frac{100}{\text{difference}} = \frac{100}{1.6} = 71$$

  Thirty-one percent of the Hux and Naylor participants would choose to take the drug given the NNT figures.
- The **disease-free survival** time is 15 weeks, and 40% of the Hux and Naylor participants would choose to take the drug based on these results.
- Hux and Naylor did not give the **cost-per-life-year-saved** data, **the number of pills needed to be taken** to prevent one additional event, or the *P*-value to the participants for assessment. The *P*-values on their own are even less helpful than some of the other numbers researchers use to present their results of their studies.

Differences in risk between study groups are most often represented as absolute differences and relative differences, with the numbers needed to treat data becoming more common with time. The absolute and relative differences are ones you have already seen in the cream cheese discussion.

Absolute Risk Difference

The absolute difference is the arithmetic difference between the rates of events in the intervention, or experimental group and the control group. It can be expressed in four different ways, depending on what is being measured (whether "good" or "bad") and whether the rates of the outcome events are increased or decreased when comparing the study groups.

An **absolute risk reduction** occurs when the risk of a bad event (for example, death, fever, myocardial infarction, or recurrence) decreases as a result of an intervention, compared with control treatment or no treatment. This is the most common type of outcome.

An **absolute benefit increase** occurs when the risk of a good event (for example, abstinence from alcohol, successful pregnancy, or base salary) increases when an intervention is compared with control treatment or no treatment.

An **absolute risk increase** occurs when the risk of a bad event (for example, breast cancer after hormone replacement therapy or gastrointestinal hemorrhage after taking aspirin to prevent strokes) increases when an intervention is compared with control treatment or no treatment.

An **absolute benefit reduction** occurs when the benefit of a good outcome decreases (for example, teaching reading skills with whole language techniques did not produce more readers by fifth grade—the control group did better than the experimental or intervention group). Few trials with these benefit reduction outcomes exist.

Relative Risk Difference

The **relative risk difference** is the proportional difference between the rates of events in the experimental group and the control group, taking into account the control group rate. Relative differences are always bigger than absolute differences, and often tend to inflate perceptions of what the results of the study truly are. Some clinicians admit using relative numbers (the larger numbers) when they want the patient to choose the treatment, and using absolute numbers (the smaller numbers) when they would like them not to.

The relative risk difference is calculated by dividing the absolute difference by the control rate; that is (experimental or intervention rate – control rate)/control rate. It can be expressed similarly to the above:

- relative risk reduction,
- relative benefit increase,
- relative risk increase, and
- relative benefit reduction.

Number Needed-to-Treat

The **number needed-to-treat (NNT)** is defined as the number of patients that one clinician would need to treat with the experimental treatment or intervention to achieve one additional patient who has a favorable response or outcome. For example, the NNT for a new anti-nausea drug for children during chemotherapy is two. This means that two children would have to be treated with the drug to have one additional child be protected from being nauseous after chemotherapy compared with what would have happened if the children had not been treated for nausea during chemotherapy. Another example is an NNT of 12,000 for mass screening of adults to determine if they have colorectal cancer. This means that 12,000 persons would need to be screened for colorectal cancer to prevent one additional death at 5 years. In summary, the smaller the NNT is, the more effective is the treatment. Although not all that easy to understand at first glance, it is a representation of the results of studies which is being used more and more frequently.

The number needed-to-treat is calculated as 100/absolute difference, and can be either "number needed-to-treat" for studies with positive results or "number needed-to-harm" for studies with negative results. For example, an NNH of 42 would mean that, for every 42 persons with rheumatoid arthritis who were treated with nonsteroidal anti-inflammatory agents, one additional person would have a major gastrointestinal hemorrhage by 2 years.

Confidence Interval

The **confidence interval** (**CI**) quantifies the uncertainty of a result or statistic. A 95% CI means the range of values within which we can be 95% sure that the number or result given falls within that range if we repeated the study. For example, a weight loss study might find that the mean difference in weight loss in the two groups was 5 kg with a 95% CI of ± 2 kg. This means that if we repeated the study 100 times the mean difference would be between 3 and 7 kg for 95% of the trials (5 ± 2).[9,10]

Calculations

One of the best ways to understand numerical presentations of data is to actually do the calculations oneself. The following data come from a well-done systematic review article by Grady et al.[11] It is a comprehensive presentation of the risks and benefits of using hormone replacement therapy (HRT) for postmenopausal women that had been proved by 1992 (some of these results have changed since then). The American College of Physicians used these data in the development of their clinical practice guideline (recommendations for consideration). The guideline was designed to provide data and discussion issues for women and clinicians to use in making the complex decision to take HRT during and after menopause.[12] The following data are for a hypothetical woman who is considering taking HRT. She has the following characteristics. The relevant statistics (lifetime probabilities) for various conditions and diseases are listed below:

- 50 years old
- White race
- No history of breast cancer
- Strong family history of cardiovascular disease
- HRT will be long-term and include estrogen and progestin taken in a cyclical pattern

Long-term hormone replacement therapy versus placebo for a 50-year-old white woman

Disease	Rate with no HRT	Rate with HRT
Coronary heart disease (CHD)	46%	34%
Stroke	20%	20%
Breast cancer	10%	13%
Endometrial cancer	3%	3%
Hip fracture	13%	15%
Life expectancy	83 years	84 years

No differences are seen in the rates of disease for stroke and endometrial cancer, so consideration of these two diseases is not an issue in the question for this woman of whether to take HRT. To gain practice with calculations use the data for CHD and breast cancer and calculate the absolute differences, the relative differences, and the numbers needed to treat or harm for this person.

Coronary Heart Disease With HRT
    Rate of CHD with no HRT (control)   _____
    Rate of CHD with HRT (experimental)   _____

      Absolute Risk   Reduction?   Increase?
                      Control rate – experimental rate

                      _____ – _____

                      = _____

      Relative Risk   Reduction?   Increase?
                      (Control rate – experimental rate)/control rate

                      (_____ – _____)/(_____)

                      = _____ / _____

                      = _____

    Number Needed-to-Treat = 100/(Control rate – experimental rate)
                      = 100/(_____)
                      = _____

Breast Cancer With HRT
    Rate of breast cancer with no HRT (control)   _____
    Rate of breast cancer with HRT (experimental)   _____

      Absolute Risk   Reduction?   Increase?
                      Control rate – experimental rate

                      _____ – _____

                      = _____

      Relative Risk   Reduction?   Increase?
                      (Control rate – experimental rate)/control rate

                      (_____ – _____)/(_____)

                      = _____ / _____

                      = _____

    Number Needed-to-Harm = 100/(Control rate – experimental rate)
                      = 100/(_____)
                      = _____

Solutions

Coronary Heart Disease With HRT

Rate of CHD with no HRT (control) _____46%_____

Rate of CHD with HRT (experimental) _____34%_____

Absolute Risk ⟨Reduction?⟩ ~~Increase?~~

Control rate – experimental rate

_____46%_____ – _____34%_____

= _____12%_____

Relative Risk ⟨Reduction?⟩ ~~Increase?~~

(Control rate – experimental rate)/control rate

(_____46%_____ – _____34%_____)/(46%)

= _____12%_____ / _____46%_____

= _____26%_____

Number Needed-to-Treat = 100/(Control rate – experimental rate)

= 100/(12)

= 8.3 rounded up to 9

Breast Cancer With HRT

Rate of breast cancer with no HRT (control) _____10%_____

Rate of breast cancer with HRT (experimental) _____13%_____

Absolute Risk ~~Reduction?~~ ⟨Increase?⟩

Control rate – experimental rate

_____10%_____ – _____13%_____

= _____3%_____ Don't worry about minus sign (negative number)

Relative Risk ~~Reduction?~~ ⟨Increase?⟩

(Control rate – experimental rate)/control rate

(_____10%_____ – _____13%_____)/(10%)

= _____3%_____ / _____10%_____

= _____30%_____

Number Needed-to-Harm = 100/(Control rate – experimental rate)

= 100/(3)

= 33.3 rounded upt to 34

Summary: For the 50-year-old woman who is considering HRT, the numbers related to *coronary heart disease* and *breast cancer* are:

CHD	Breast cancer
Absolute risk reduction—12%	Absolute risk increase—3%
Relative risk reduction—26%	Relative risk increase—30%
NNT—8.3 or 9	NNH—33.3 or 34

These are the data that I used in my decision to take HRT. I looked at the data, especially the raw rates of occurrences in the table and also the NNT and NNH values. I also took my family history into account: my mother and both grandmothers died of heart problems, as did many other relatives. Adding in the symptoms of menopause, I chose to start taking HRT, and I have not regretted my decision. I will remain open, however, to data from large, randomized controlled trials of HRT that are now being done. Some initial evidence from them says that the data used here for CHD protection might be a high estimate of the true worth of HRT in cardiovascular disease. Some epidemiologists are saying that evidence may show that women who choose to take HRT are inherently more healthy as opposed to the situation that HRT produces healthier women.

Summary

Therapy, prevention and control, and quality improvement studies use a randomized controlled trial study design. Important aspects of the studies are the randomization, blinding, and follow-up. The Evidence-Based Medicine Working Group at McMaster has produced a series of *Reader's Guides* for clinicians and others to use in reading and evaluating the articles for clinical application. A full listing of the series is in the appendix, and the articles themselves are on the Internet at http: *//hiru.mcmaster.ca/ebm/ default.htm.* The ranked list of the clinical importance of therapy design characteristics in evaluating the articles for making patient care decisions (steps three and four of the EBHC process) is as follows:[13]

- Randomization (properly done, of course)
- Follow up (80% is the goal for strong research).
- Blind (triple-is best, followed by double-and then single-blinding).
- Proved baseline similarities at the start of the trial.
- Large numerical differences between the study groups at the end of the trial.

These features constitute a well-done therapy study. A fuller description of clinical trials is included in a recent book by Jadad.[14] The next step is to examine how indexers who produce the four databases index for the study methodology. Both index terms and the terms and phrases authors use in their titles and abstracts (called **textwords**) can be used to construct search strategies. After the tables for MEDLINE, CINAHL, PsycINFO, and EMBASE/Excerpta Medica, several examples of research studies are included, with indexing and textwords related to methodology highlighted. Examining the indexing and author use of methods terms can help us understand how best to retrieve randomized controlled trials from the literature.

For those without strong database searching skills, the material in Chapter 1 includes some hints on searching. Most searching systems have built-in tutorials. Librarians are also good sources of information or training.

MEDLINE

Index Terms, Publication Types, and Textwords for Therapy Trials

Medical Subject Headings (MeSH)
Research
    Clinical protocols
    Feasibility studies
    Pilot studies
    Reproducibility of results
        Research design
            Double-blind method
            Meta-analysis
            Patient selection
            Random allocation
            Sample size

Epidemiologic research design
    Crossover studies
    Double-blind method*
    Matched pair analysis
    Meta-analysis
    Random allocation
    Reproducibility of results
    Sample size
    Sensitivity and specificity
    Seroepidemiologic methods
    Single-blind method

Clinical trials
    Clinical trials, phase I
    Clinical trials, phase II
    Clinical trials, phase III
    Clinical trials, phase IV
    Controlled clinical trials
    Multicenter trials
    Randomized controlled trials

Placebos*

Comparative study

Outcome assessment (health care)
Treatment outcome
Medical futility
Treatment failure

Publication Types
Clinical trial*
Clinical trial, phase I
Clinical trial, phase II
Clinical trial, phase III
Clinical trial, phase IV
Controlled clinical trial
Randomized controlled trial*
Multicenter study
Meta-analysis

Subheadings
Therapy
Surgery
Radiotherapy
Diet therapy
Nursing
Psychology
Therapeutic use
Drug therapy
Rehabilitation
Chemically induced

Textwords
Random:*
Single-blind:
Double-blind:
Triple-blind:
Double-dummy
Mask:
Sham
Placebo:*
Control: trial:
Efficacy (can it work in an ideal world?)
Effectiveness (can it work in a real world?)

---

*indicates a preferred term

The designation ":" after a term or phrase is a truncation indication. This means that the textword, "random:" would pick up all words that included the six letters and alternate endings (for example, random, randomized, randomised, randomly, and so on).

Notes on Terms in MEDLINE

Note that with the introduction of publication types in 1990–1991 major changes have occurred in indexing for methodology for therapy studies. Some MeSH terms such as "Randomized controlled trials" (MeSH), have actually changed meanings in the transition to publication types. MeSH indexing indicates articles that are "about" the specific MeSH heading. For example, the MeSH term, "Clinical trials" is used when an author writes about the history of clinical trials, describes how to do a certain aspect of clinical trials, such as blinding, or is using clinical trials in producing a systematic review article. Publication types describe what something "is"—for example, an obituary, a bibliography, a review article, a clinical trial, or a randomized controlled trial. Where "dual" terms exist as MeSH and publication types, often the MeSH is in a plural form, and the publication type is in the singular form.

Note also that indexers are not consistent with their assignment of MeSH headings and this was shown elegantly in the study by Funk et al.[15] Their results can be extrapolated to other databases: you will get better retrieval by combining several index terms and textwords with "ORs" and trying various combinations of the terms, depending on the topic and need.

CINAHL Database of Nursing and Allied Health Literature

CINAHL Index Terms and Documentation Types for Therapy Trials

CINAHL Index Terms
Research methodology
    Data analysis
        Meta-analysis
    Data collection
    Sampling methods
    Study design
        Crossover design
        Empirical research
            Experimental studies
                Clinical trials*
                    Double-blind studies
                    Intervention studies
                    Prevention trials
                    Single-blind studies
                    Therapeutic studies
                    Triple-blind studies

Clinical research
    Clinical nursing research

Comparative studies

Random assignment

Reproducibility of results (Health care)

Outcomes (Health care)
    Medical futility
    Nursing outcomes
    Outcome assessment
    Outcomes of prematurity
    Pregnancy outcomes
    Treatment outcomes
        Treatment failure

Placebos

Patient selection

Professional practice, research based
    Nursing practice, research based

Random sample
    Simple random sample
    Stratified random sample
    Systematic random sample

Sample size

CINAHL Subheadings
Prevention and control
Therapeutic use
Therapy
Nursing
Evaluation
Rehabilitation
Drug therapy
Surgery
Radiotherapy
Diet therapy

CINAHL Documentation Types
Research*
Clinical trial*
Tables/charts
Nursing interventions
Protocol

Textwords
Random:*
Single-blind:
Double-blind:
Triple-blind:
Double-dummy
Mask:
Sham
Placebo:*
Control: trial:
Efficacy (can it work in an ideal world?)
Effectiveness (can it work in a real world?)

---

*indicates a preferred term
CINAHL thesaurus terms selected by Katy Nesbit
All extracts from the CINAHL® Thesaurus Copyright © 1999, Cinahl Information Systems. Reprinted with permission from Cinahl Information Systems.

PsycINFO

(used with permission American Psychological Association)

Index Terms for Therapy Trials

Methodology Descriptors and Publication Types

Methodology (Definition: Conceptually broad array term that refers generally to strategies, techniques or procedures used in applied, descriptive, or experimental studies. Used for Research Methods)

  Cohort Analysis
  Data Collection
  Empirical Methods + (Note: many clinical trials seem to be indexed to this term)
    Experimental Methods
    Observation Methods
  Meta Analysis

Experimental Design (Definition: General procedural plan for conducting an experiment in view of the specific data desired. This may include identification of the independent and dependent variables; selection of subjects and their assignment to specific experimental conditions/treatments; the sequence of experimental conditions/treatments; and a method of analysis. Used for Design (experimental) and Research design).

  Between Groups Design
  Cohort Analysis

Follow-up Studies
Longitudinal Studies
Repeated Measures

Experimental Subjects
Experiment Volunteers

Experiment Controls (Used for Control groups)

Experimental Replication

Sampling (Experimental)
Biased Sampling
Random Sampling

Placebo

Treatment Outcomes+
Psychotherapeutic Outcomes

Treatment Effectiveness Evaluation

Publication Type or Form/Content Type
Empirical Study (Note: Many trials seem to be indexed to this publication type)
Experimental Replication
Followup Study
Longitudinal Study
Meta Analysis
Prospective Study
Retrospective Study
Treatment Outcome Study

Textwords
Clinical protocol:*
Feasability stud:*
Pilot stud:*
Randomized controlled trial*
Random:*
Double blind:*
Double dummy
Masked
Sham
Clinical trial:*
Controlled trial:*
Controlled clinical trial:*
Multicenter study
Comparative stud:*

Outcome:* assessment
Efficacy
Effectiveness

Notes on Terms in PsycINFO

PsycINFO presents a challenge to those searching for EBHC topics. Unlike MEDLINE, it does not include subheadings which may be attached to descriptors, or free-floated in order to narrow, broaden, or otherwise refine retrieval. Also note that methodology descriptors can indicate that the citation is about the technique or it can indicate the "form" of the research.

However, the database does have descriptors which are roughly the conceptual equivalent of MeSH Subheadings. Many of these are broad headings, such as "treatment" (used for therapy), and may be exploded or used in addition to include retrieval from more specific descriptors. Note: The explosion function in your vendor's version of PsycINFO may differ in its mechanics from the explosion function in MEDLINE. Consult your database vendor for specifics.

Descriptors used in this section were taken from the Thesaurus of Psychological Index Terms, Seventh Edition. This is a suggested list of descriptors, and we recommend that you consult your thesaurus for additional terms for concepts such as drugs, disorders, or tests.

+ indicated other terms that can be exploded
*indicates a preferred term
PsycINFO terms selected by Jean Sullivant

EMBASE/EXCERPTA MEDICA

Index Terms, Links, and EMTAGS for Therapy Trials

Index terms

Controlled study
   Case control study
   Randomized controlled trial

Drug comparison

Clinical trial* (do not use Clinical study)
   Multicenter study
   Phase 1 clinical trial
   Phase 2 clinical trial
   Phase 3 clinical trial
   Phase 4 clinical trial
   Randomized controlled trial*

Major clinical study*

Medical research
    Cancer research
    Clinical research
    Drug research
    Gerontological research

Evidence based medicine
    Meta-analysis
    Outcomes research
    Randomized controlled trial

Randomization
Cross-over procedure
Double blind procedure
Single blind procedure
Placebo

Links (subheadings)
Clinical trial
Drug comparison*
Drug therapy
Prevention
Radiotherapy
Rehabilitation
Surgery
Therapy [does not include drug therapy, ratiotherapy, or surgery]

Emtags (publication types)
Major clinical study [at least 50 patients studied]
Clinical studies [use for clinical studies before 1978 and limited to "significant
    studies for 1978 to 1986]
Clinical article [studies of 5 to 49 patients]
Controlled study [studies with a control group]
Prevention
Therapy

---

*indicates a preferred term

MEDLINE HEDGES

In 1992, the U.S. National Library of Medicine provided research funds for the evaluation of retrieval terms (index and author textwords) for randomized controlled trials and also for diagnosis, etiology and causation, and prognosis and natural history articles. Several thousand proposed single-term or complex, multiterm search strategies for retrieval were compared against a hand search. The hand search categorized all articles in

10 selected medical and internal medicine journals for 1986 and 1991 for methodologies such as randomized controlled trials. The study results are reported in an article by Haynes et al.[16] Although the search strategies are probably dated because of changing indexing practices and changes in presentation of trial results since 1992, the "best" single-term strategy for MEDLINE that retrieves the least irrelevant material in a search for therapy, prevention and control, and quality improvement articles is:

clinical trial (publication type)

The "best" complex or multiterm strategy for MEDLINE that retrieves the smallest amount of irrelevant material for therapy, prevention and control, and quality improvement is:

randomized controlled trial (publication type)

OR drug therapy (MeSH)

OR therapeutic use (MeSH)

OR all random: (textword)

The best possible search strategy that retrieves the most relevant and high-quality articles is:

all double blind: (textword)

OR all placebo: (textword)

This research will, it is hoped, be updated in 1999 and be extended to include retrievals for CINAHL, PsycINFO, and EMBASE. No high quality, studies to evaluate and validate searching strategies in CINAHL, PsycINFO, or EMBASE have been reported. The strategies above, termed by librarians as "hedges," are also embedded in PubMed, an Internet-based MEDLINE service from the U.S. National Library of Medicine, as "clinical queries." Hedges are to be used in conjunction with content-based searching. For example, a search on using chewing gum that contains the artificial sugar, xylitol, for reducing otitis media or cavities in children could be done using the content (xylitol AND chewing gum) ANDed with any of the "hedges" above to limit retrieval to citations that have strong evidence value (clinical trials).

Examples of MEDLINE Indexing and Textwords

One of the best ways to learn how to search is to check how indexers have indexed studies similar to the ones you would like to retrieve. Here are some examples from MEDLINE.

Example 2–1
Burke GS, Lapidus GD, Zavoski RW, et al. Evaluation of the effectiveness of a pavement stencil in promoting safe behavior among elementary school children boarding school buses. Pediatrics 1996;97:520–3.

This study is a randomized controlled trial designed to improve school bus boarding safety. Nine school bus stops met the inclusion criteria: children attended any one of four elementary schools; children were from kindergarten to sixth grade; all children lived more than one mile from the school; more than nine children regularly waited at the school bus stop; and the waiting area was paved. Five bus stops were randomly allocated to have a yellow school bus stencil painted on the sidewalk for the children to wait behind, and four bus stops were allocated to have the children wait in areas related to the natural geography of the area (behind hedges, sidewalk cracks, and so on). For 5 weeks parent volunteers measured the safety behavior of the children. Children who waited using the yellow stencil were less likely to leave the safety area than those who did not have a stencil to wait behind.

Issues From This Study

- Bus stops, not people, were randomized.
- Blinding not possible for any group (children, bus drivers, or parent volunteer assessors).
- Sample sizes do not have to be equal.
- Can do simple numbers (number or proportion of students who act safely).
- Can do complex analyses (factor in the number of boys who wait at each stop if the groups were not equal for the number of boys and girls.)

Retrieval Strategy Can Use Any of the Following:

MeSH indexing   Evaluation studies
Textwords   Effectiveness (title and abstract)
                      Randomly assigned (abstract)
                      Cost-effective (abstract)
                      Odds ratio (abstract)

Note: the indexers at NLM did not index as a clinical trial (publication type) as this article does not fit their definition of a clinical trial—more of a clinical slant is needed before the indexers will use the term clinical trial (publication type).

Example 2–2
Maizels M, Scott B, Cohen W, Chen W. Intranasal lidocaine for treatment of migraine: a randomized, double-blind, controlled trial. JAMA 1996;276:319–21.

This study was done to assess the effectiveness (does it work in the real world?) of intranasal lidocaine to reduce headache pain in adults with migraine. Eighty-one patients from California were studied. Inclusion criteria were patients who were more than 18 years old, patients had migraine headache with or without aura defined using

MEDLINE Record for Example 2–1

Unique Identifier   96211675

Authors   Burke GS. Lapidus GD. Zavoski RW. Wallace L. Banco LI.

Institution   Connecticut Childhood Injury Prevention Center, Hartford Hospital, Connecticut 06102-5037, USA.

Title   Evaluation of the **effectiveness** of a pavement stencil in promoting safe behavior among elementary school children boarding school buses.

Source   Pediatrics. 97(4):520–3, 1996 Apr.

MeSH Subject Headings
*Accidents, Traffic/pc [Prevention & Control]   Human
Child   Male
*Child Behavior   *Motor Vehicles
Child, Preschool   *Safety
Evaluation Studies   *Schools
Female

Abstract
OBJECTIVE: The majority of school bus-related fatalities among children attending elementary school in the United States occur as children board or alight from buses. Injuries occur during boarding when children enter the street and are struck by buses or other vehicles. This study evaluated the **effectiveness** of a stencil in the shape of a school bus applied to the pavement at a bus stop in improving safe behaviors at bus stops. Specifically, we assessed the frequency of children running toward the bus as it approached or entered the street. METHODS: Elementary school bus stops with similar roadways, traffic profiles, and numbers of children boarding participated in the study. Stops were **randomly assigned** to an intervention group, in which children were instructed to remain within a safe area during boarding that was demarcated by a pavement stencil, or an education-only group, in which the safe area was demarcated by some existing environmental feature. Both groups received education about safe boarding procedures. Observers rated behavior at each stop daily for 5 consecutive weeks. Data were analyzed as bivariate odds of any unsafe behavior in the education-only group. RESULTS: One hundred forty-five observations from seven bus stops with stencils and 174 daily observations from six education-only stops were completed. Observations of children in the education-only group were twice as likely to show unsafe behavior while waiting (**odds ratio** [OR], 2.1; 95% confidence inter-val [CI], 1.3–3.6) and during boarding (OR, 2.1; 95% CI, 1.2-3.9). ORs were significantly higher in the education-only group for boys, girls, and children in grades 4 through 6. When no adult was present, there was a greater likelihood of unsafe behavior among all children in the education-only group while waiting (OR, 16.1; 95% CI, 3.9-72.4) and during boarding (OR, 15.0; 95% CI, 3.2–81.4).The presence of an adult at the stop did not have an independent effect on behavior. Children at education-only stops located on roadways with high traffic volume were more likely to engage in unsafe behavior while waiting (OR, 8.0; 95% CI, 3.8–17.3) and during boarding (OR, 4.9; 95% CI, 2.2–11.0). No differences were observed during boarding between stencil and education-only groups when 10 or more children were at the stops. CONCLUSION: The pavement stencil, when accompanied by education about safe boarding, may represent a **cost-effective** approach to reducing unsafe behavior at bus stops by children of elementary school age.

Publication Type   Journal Article.

the International Headache Society classification, current headache of at least moderate severity and lasting for less than 3 days, headache frequency less than 1 per week, and no allergy to lidocaine. Fifty-three patients were randomly allocated to intranasal lidocaine (4% solution), and 28 patients were randomly allocated to a saline placebo. Outcomes were a reduction in headache pain of 50% or more within 15 minutes of nasal spray assessed in a blinded fashion (double-blinding); reduction in nausea and photophobia; relapse of migraine; and change in disability scores. At 15 minutes the rate of pain reduction 50% or more was 55% in the lidocaine group and 21% in the placebo group. Reviewing some of the statistics we have looked at, the study results can be represented as:

- Absolute benefit increase (pain reduction) (difference—55%–21%) = 34%.
- Relative benefit increase (difference/baseline rate = 34%/21%) = 162%.
- NNT = 100/absolute difference = 100/34 = 3

Issues From this Study

- Many ways to present the results of the study.
- Groups were dissimilar in size—done on purpose to keep the number of persons who received salt solution for their headache to a minimum.
- Good, consistent indexing and textword use.

Retrieval Strategy Can Use Any of the Following:

MeSH indexing	Clinical trial (publication type)
	Randomized controlled trial (publication type)
	Double-blind method (MeSH)
	Prospective studies
	Time factors
Textwords	Randomized (title, abstract)
	Double-blind (title, abstract)
	Controlled trial (title, abstract)
	Placebo (abstract)

Example 2–3
Sharpe M, Hawton K, Simkin S, et al. Cognitive behaviour therapy for the chronic fatigue syndrome: a randomised controlled trial. BMJ 1996;312:22–6.

Of 123 patients with chronic fatigue syndrome, 60 were entered into the study. All received standard medical care. Thirty patients received extra encouragement to exercise, and 30 received 16 one-hour cognitive behavioral therapy sessions run by experienced therapists. All patients were assessed at 4 months, and the outcome was normal functioning. The rate of normal functioning was higher in patients in the cognitive

MEDLINE Record for Example 2–2

Unique Identifier   96286145

Authors   Maizels M. Scott B. Cohen W. Chen W.

Institution   Department of Family Practice, Southern California Permanente Medical Group, Woodland Hills, CA 91365, USA.

Title   Intranasal lidocaine for treatment of migraine: a randomized, **double-blind**, controlled trial [see comments].

Source   JAMA. 276(4):319–21, 1996 Jul 24–31.

MeSH Subject Headings
Acute Disease
Administration, Intranasal
Adult
Aged
Double-Blind Method
Female
Ganglia, Parasympathetic
Human
Lidocaine/ad [Administration & Dosage]
*Lidocaine/tu [Therapeutic Use]
Male

Middle Age
*Migraine/dt [Drug Therapy]
Migraine/pp [Physiopathology]
Nausea
Palate
Prospective Studies
Recurrence
Severity of Illness Index
Sphenoid Bone
Time Factors

Abstract
OBJECTIVE: To evaluate the effectiveness of intranasal lidocaine for treatment of acute migraine headache. DESIGN: Prospective, **randomized, double-blind, placebo-controlled trial**. SETTING: Community urgent care department. PATIENTS: A total of 81 patients (67 women and 14 men; median age, 42 years; range, 19-68 years) with a chief complaint of headache who fulfilled criteria of the International Headache Society for migraine participated. Patients were excluded if headache had lasted more than 3 days or if the frequency of severe headache was more than once per week. INTERVENTION: Patients were **randomized** in a 2:1 ratio to receive a 4 percent solution of intranasal lidocaine or saline placebo, respectively. MAIN OUTCOME MEASURES: The primary outcome measure was at least 50 percent reduction of headache within 15 minutes after treatment. Secondary measures include reduction in nausea and photophobia, use of rescue medication, relapse of headache, and change in headache disability scores. RESULTS: Of 53 patients who received intranasal lidocaine, 29 (55 percent) had at least a 50 percent reduction of headache compared with 6 (21 percent) of 28 controls (P=.004). Nausea and photophobia were significantly reduced (P=.03 and P=.001, respectively). Rescue medication for headache relief was needed in 15 (28 percent) of 53 patients in the lidocaine group vs 20 (71 percent) of 28 controls (P<.001). Among those with initial relief of headache, relapse of headache occurred in 10 (42 percent) of 24 in the lidocaine group vs 5 (83 percent) of 6 in the control group (P=.17), usually within the first hour after treatment. CONCLUSIONS: Intranasal lidocaine provides rapid relief of headache in approximately 55 percent of ambulatory patients with migraine. Relapse of headache is common and occurs early after treatment.

Publication Type   Clinical Trial. Journal Article. **Randomized Controlled Trial.**

behavior group than in the usual care and exercise group (73% versus 27%). The study results can be represented as

- Absolute benefit increase (difference—73%–27%) = 46%.
- Relative benefit increase (difference/baseline rate) = 46%/27%) = 170%.
- NNT = 100/difference =100/46 = 2.3 or 3 when rounded up to a full person

Issues From This Study

- Blinding not possible, so effort was concentrated on measurement of outcomes.
- Note British spellings
- Good indexing

Retrieval Strategy Can Use Any of the Following:

MeSH indexing	Clinical trial (publication type)
	Controlled clinical trial (publication type)
	Treatment outcome (MeSH)
Textwords	Randomized (title, abstract)
	Intention to treat analysis (abstract)
	Efficacy (abstract)

Take care when using textwords for retrieving articles with methodology words. First be aware of differences in U.S. and U.K. spellings, especially terms like *randomized* and *randomised*. Similarly, be careful of differences in national usage of terms: *double-blind* in North America and *sham* and *double-dummy* in Europe. Third, be careful of terms that sound similar: for example, *a random population* often means a group of people chosen with no real method in mind, such as 100 people found at a shopping mall or a hospital clinic. Fourth, authors who use negatives to describe their study can cause retrieval of studies that are not relevant. For example, Mercado et al. say that their study is "prospective, controlled, and not randomized."[17] Use of the textword phrase "random:" will retrieve this study.

ASSIGNMENT

Answer these four questions using MEDLINE and/or CINAHL. Try to use at least some of the methods terms listed above. Suggested Search Strategies are on the CD-ROM disk.
1. Are zinc supplements beneficial for infants and small children with diarrhea?
2. Ten years ago, few drugs were available that helped patients with congestive heart failure. What are some of the new drugs, and how effective are they at reducing mortality?
3. Can sucrose be used as an analgesic for newborn infants who are having painful procedures such as heel sticks or circumcision?
4. Should persons with mild asthma take albuterol according to a regular schedule or on an "as needed" basis?

MEDLINE Record for Example 2–3

Unique Identifier   96135915

Authors   Sharpe M. Hawton K. Simkin S. Surawy C. Hackmann A. Klimes I. Peto T. Warrell D. Seagroatt V.

Institution   University Department of Psychiatry, Warneford Hospital, Oxford.

Title   Cognitive behaviour therapy for the chronic fatigue syndrome: a **randomised controlled trial** [see comments].

Source   BMJ. 312(7022):22–6, 1996 Jan 6.

MeSH Subject Headings
Adaptation, Psychological	Female
Adult	Human
Attitude to Health	Male
*Cognitive Therapy	Patient Compliance
Depression/co [Complications]	Support, Non-U.S. Gov't
Fatigue Syndrome, Chronic/px [Psychology]	**Treatment Outcome**
*Fatigue Syndrome, Chronic/th [Therapy]	

Abstract
OBJECTIVE: To evaluate the acceptability and efficacy of adding cognitive behaviour therapy to the medical care of patients presenting with the chronic fatigue syndrome. DESIGN: Randomised controlled trial with final assessment at 12 months. SETTING: An infectious diseases outpatient clinic. SUBJECTS: 60 consecutively referred patients meeting consensus criteria for the chronic fatigue syndrome. INTERVENTIONS: Medical care comprised assessment, advice, and follow up in general practice. Patients who received cognitive behaviour therapy were offered 16 individual weekly sessions in addition to their medical care. MAIN OUTCOME MEASURES: The proportions of patients (a) who achieved normal daily functioning (Karnofsky score 80 or more) and (b) who achieved a clinically significant improvement in functioning (change in Karnofsky score 10 points or more) by 12 months after randomisation. RESULTS: Only two eligible patients refused to participate. All randomised patients completed treatment. An intention to treat analysis showed that 73% (22/30) of recipients of cognitive behaviour therapy achieved a satisfactory outcome as compared with 27% (8/30) of patients who were given only medical care (difference 47 percentage points; 95% confidence interval 24 to 69). Similar differences were observed in subsidiary outcome measures. The improvement in disability among patients given cognitive behaviour therapy continued after completion of therapy. Illness beliefs and coping behaviour previously associated with a poor outcome changed more with cognitive behaviour therapy than with medical care alone. CONCLUSION: Adding cognitive behaviour therapy to the medical care of patients with the chronic fatigue syndrome is acceptable to patients and leads to a sustained reduction in functional impairment.

Publication Type   **Clinical Trial.** Journal Article. **Randomized Controlled Trial.**

This article was first published in the BMJ 1996 Jan 6; 312:22–6 and is reproduced with permission of the BMJ.

REFERENCES

1. Dubois JM, Bartter T, Pratter MR. Music improves patients comfort level during outpatient bronchoscopy. Chest 1995;108:129–30.
2. Maizels H, Scott B, Cohen W, Chen W. Intranasal lidocaine for treatment of migraine. A randomized, double-blind, controlled trial. JAMA 1996;276:319–21.
3. Hemila H. Vitamin C, the placebo effects, and the common cold. A case study of how preconceptions influence the analysis of results. J Clin Epidemiol 1996;49:1079–84.
4. Christakis GT, Lichtenstein SV, Buth KJ, et al. The influence of risk on the results of warm heart surgery: a substudy of a randomized trial. Eur J Cardiothorac Surg 1997;11:515–20.
5. Chaput de Saintonge DM, Cross KW, Shathorn MK, et al. Hats for the newborn infant. BMJ 1979;2:570–1.
6. Gwon A. Topical ofloxacin compared with gentamicin in the treatment of external ocular infection. Ofloxacin Study Group. Br J Ophthalmol 1992;76:714–8.
7. Frick MH, Elo O, Haapa K, et al. Helinski heart study: primary-prevention trial with gemfibrozil in middle-aged men with dyslipidemia. N Engl J Med 1987;317:1237–45.
8. Hux JE, Naylor CD. Communicating the benefits of chronic preventive therapy: does the format of efficacy determine patients acceptance of treatment. Med Decis Making 1995;15:152–7.
9. Altman DG. Evidence-based medicine. 1996;1:164–6.
10. Glossary. Evidence-based nursing. 1998;1:inside back cover.
11. Grady D, Rubin SM, Petitti DB, et al. Hormone therapy to prevent disease and prolong life in postmenopausal women. Ann Intern Med 1992;117:1016–37.
12. American College of Physicians. Guidelines for counseling postmenopausal women about preventive hormone therapy. Ann Intern Med 1992;117:1038–41.
13. Guyatt GH, Sackett DL, Cook DJ for the Evidence-Based Medicine Working Group. Users' guides to the medical literature. II. How to use an article about therapy or prevention. A. Are the results of the study valid? JAMA 1993;270:2598–601.
14. Jadad AR. Randomized controlled trials. A user's guide. London: BMJ Books; 1998.
15. Funk ME, Reid DA. Indexing consistency in MEDLINE. Bull Med Libr Assoc 1983:71:278–84.
16. Haynes RB, Wilczynski NL, McKibbon KA, et al. Developing optimal search strategies for detecting clinically sound studies in MEDLINE. J Am Med Inform Assoc 1994;1:447–58.
17. Mercado MA, Horales-Linares JC, Granados-Garcia J, et al. Distal splenorenal shunt versus 10-mm low-diameter mesocaval shunt for variceal hemorrhage. Am J Surg 1996;171:591–5.

3

Diagnosis and Screening

The category of therapy has the most publications of any of the categories of health care research. The second most common type of research is diagnosis. Health professionals are always looking for better ways to determine if diseases or conditions are present in both symptomatic (diagnosis) and asymptomatic (screening) patients. Clinicians and researchers define better diagnostic or screening tests as ones that give more accurate results faster, and at a lower cost in terms of safety, comfort, and expense.

CLINICAL EXAMPLE: FAST, ACCURATE DIAGNOSIS OF HUMAN IMMUNODEFICIENCY VIRUS INFECTION

As with the previous chapter, we will start with an example of a problem and the research that went into solving it. The problem was that AIDS/HIV tests results take 1 to 2 weeks before the resulting diagnosis can be given to a patient. Montefiore Hospital in the Bronx, New York has one of the highest incidences of HIV infection in North America.[1] It also has a large transient patient population. So even if patients consent to be tested, would they come back in weeks for the test results? The hospital staff wanted to find a faster test for HIV infection than the usual Western blot test. They identified an ELISA enzyme test that takes 10 minutes for the results to be known. The next step was to compare it with the usual test, the Western blot test.

Eight hundred and thirty-seven patients with unknown HIV status were tested. Each of the patients received both the ELISA test *and* the Western blot test. The technicians or clinicians who read the ELISA test results did not know the results of the Western blot testing, and the laboratory personnel who did the Western blot testing did not know the results of the ELISA tests. The two sets of test results were compared for agreements: pairs of test results were both positive or both negative. Forty-five patients (5%) had HIV infection, and only nine pairs of samples had different test results (positive/negative pair or negative/positive pair). Because of the strong agreement between the tests and the speed of getting results from the ELISA kits, the ELISA test is now the test of choice for HIV infection at Montefiore Hospital.

HOW A DIAGNOSIS STUDY IS DONE

The best procedure for evaluating a new diagnostic or screening test involves gathering a group of persons and administering the tests that are to be evaluated. This group should include persons with different disease severities (that is, some without, some with moderate, and some with severe disease). *Each* person must undergo *both* a currently used **gold standard** procedure (often also called the **diagnostic standard** or **criterion standard**) and a new, it is hoped better, test. Often, the standard test is invasive (for example, surgery or an autopsy to check for the presence of stomach cancer), expensive (for example, a night in a sleep laboratory to evaluate sleep apnea), or time consuming (for example, a week to culture bronchial lavage fluid to determine whether a patient in the intensive care unit has tuberculosis). The interpretation, or reading, of the gold or diagnostic standard should be done without knowledge of the new test **and** the interpretation of the new test should be done without knowledge of the gold or diagnostic standard test.

Diagnostic tests are used for persons who have signs and symptoms that make clinicians suspicious of the presence of a specific disease or several possible diseases (for example, cough can indicate a cold, lung cancer, whooping cough, or an adverse reaction to some antihypertension medications). Screening tests are done for persons who have no clinical signs or symptoms for the disease tested for (for example, mammographies to detect breast cancer in all women over the age of 50 years). Both diagnostic and screening tests are evaluated using the same testing methodology, and the results are presented using the same terminology and statistics. "Good" tests are ones that give positive results when the disease or condition is present *and* give negative results when the disease or condition is absent. Measures of the "positive-when-should-be-positive" and "negative-when-should-be-negative" are called the **test characteristics**, and are described below. Briefly, they are, sensitivity and specificity; positive and negative predictive values; positive and negative likelihood ratios; and false positive and false negative rates.

2 X 2 TABLE

Often, data from the evaluation of a screening or diagnostic test are presented in a 2 × 2 table (or 2 by 2). The **"truth"** or gold standard results go across the top of the table, and the new test results go down the left hand side of the table. Pictorially it has the following structure, with the boxes, or **data cells**, labeled *a, b, c,* and *d.* For example, in the 2 × 2 table below, the number of persons listed in box or cell *a* is the number of persons who have a positive test result using the gold standard test *and* a positive test result using the new test being evaluated. Cell *a* can also be called the **number of true positives.** Cell *d* is the number of true negatives, cell *b* is the number of false positives, and cell *c* is the number of false negatives. Data in the four cells *a* through *d* are used to calculate the test characteristics.

Disease/condition (gold standard)
Positive   Negative
    +   –

New test + positive results	a	b	a+b
New test – negative results	c	d	c+d
	a+c	b+d	a+b+c+d

Sensitivity = a/(a + c)
Specificity = d/(b + d)

Positive likelihood ratio = sensitivity/(100 – specificity)
Negative likelihood ratio = (100 – sensitivity)/specificity

Positive predictive value = a/(a + b)
Negative predictive value = d/(c + d)

False positive rate = 100 – specificity *or* b/(b + d)
False negative rate = 100 – sensitivity *or* c/(a + c)

DEFINITIONS

The testing of diagnostic procedures initially looks fairly straight forward. It is, however, the clinical research methodology that has the most jargon. Researchers compare the results of the old (or gold) test (positive and negative) with the results of the new test (positive and negative). They want to make sure the new test results are correct as often as possible: i.e., positive when they should be positive *and* negative when they should be negative.

Sensitivity and Specificity

The two most frequently used measures of this correctness are the sensitivity and specificity of the test. Sensitivity measures the proportion of patients with the disease or disorder who have a positive result. The standard pregnancy test based on biochemical analysis of hormone levels has a high sensitivity (Table 3–1). It detects correctly a large proportion of the patients who are pregnant. Using the data from the table, the new test has a sensitivity of 98% (calculated using the formula a/(a+c) or 23/25).

The specificity of the test measures the proportion of patients without the disorder or condition who have a negative test result. The standard biochemical pregnancy test

Table 3–1
Example Using Data Comparing Pregnancy Tests of 100 Women

	Pregnancy (test repeated over time)					
	Positive +		Negative −			
New test + positive results	23	a	b	0	a + b	23
New test − negative results	2	c	d	75	c + d	77
	25	a + c	b + d	75	a + b + c + d	100

has a very high specificity. It rules out pregnancy if a woman is not pregnant—in other words, the test results would not be positive if a woman was not pregnant. The specificity for the pregnancy test is 100% (calculated using the formula d/(c+d) or 75/75).

Both sensitivity and specificity must be high for a diagnostic test to be truly useful in a clinical setting. In practice, both sensitivity and specificity should be over 80% for a clinically useful test. For screening tests such as prostate-specific antigen test to detect prostate cancer in asymptomatic men, the performance should be close to perfect (100%) to avoid incorrectly diagnosing people without the disorder, whereas diagnostic tests can function well with a lesser sensitivity and specificity. No test has a sensitivity *and* a specificity of 100%. Often, if the test result level is adjusted to maximize the sensitivity, the specificity will fall, and if the result level is changed to maximize the specificity, the sensitivity will fall.

POSITIVE PREDICTIVE VALUE AND NEGATIVE PREDICTIVE VALUE

Other measures of the "worth" or performance of a diagnostic or screening test are the positive predictive value and the negative predictive value. These are measures of what either a positive or negative test actually tells us about the probability of disease or disorder in question for the specific setting in which the test was evaluated. **Positive predictive** value is the proportion of patients with positive test results who have the disease or condition evaluated. **Negative predictive value** is the proportion of patients with negative test results who do not have the target disease or condition. The positive predictive value of the new pregnancy test for the 100 women in our sample is very high at 100% (calculated using the formula a/(a+b) or 23/23); if the test result is positive, a woman almost certainly is pregnant. The test has a smaller negative predictive value at 98% (calculated using the formula d/(d+c) or 75/77). A negative test may be negative because a woman is truly not pregnant, or simply because her reproductive system has not had enough time to produce sufficient hormone levels to test positive.

Predictive values are affected by the **prevalence** of the target disorder in the population being studied. For diagnostic test evaluation, prevalence is the proportion of patients with the target disorder among all tested patients. Prevalence is also sometimes called **pretest probability** or **pretest likelihood** of the target disorder, disease, or condition.

An example concerning pulmonary embolism illustrates the effect of prevalence on predictive values of two different populations of patients with different pretest likelihoods for pulmonary embolism. One group includes elderly patients who developed pleuritic chest pain after a complete hip replacement and who had not been given prophylactic anticoagulants to prevent blood clots. These blood clots can lead to pulmonary embolism or deep venous thrombosis, which can be fatal. The second group includes young men with similar chest pain that developed while they were playing baseball. Even though the tests these persons receive would have identical sensitivity and specificity values, the positive and negative predictive values would be different, because the pretest likelihood (prevalence) of pulmonary embolism would be much higher in elderly patients after surgery than in young men after baseball.

LIKELIHOOD RATIO

Likelihood ratios, both positive and negative (+LR and –LR), are other measures of a test's worth or performance. They indicate how much the probability of disease changes from baseline when the test result is positive (+LR) or negative (–LR). Positive likelihood ratios are taken seriously when they are in the range of 2 or more, and are clinically useful when they are greater than 5. For negative likelihood ratios the numbers for consideration are less than 0.1. A fuller explanation of the usefulness of likelihood ratios is contained in an editorial by Sackett and Straus.[2]

A test with a +LR of 24 means that a positive test result is 24 times more likely to have come from a person with the disorder of interest than from a person without the disorder. In interpreting the test results for a specific patient, a clinician must take into account how likely he or she thinks the person who is sent for testing is to have the disease or condition before testing and then apply this pretest likelihood to the final test results and published likelihood ratios for the test using a standard nomogram.

The new pregnancy test we are considering has a +LR of infinity (calculated as sensitivity/(100 – specificity) or 98/(100 – 100): any woman who has a positive test is infinitely more likely to be pregnant than if she had received a negative test result. The –LR of 0.02 (calculated as (100 – sensitivity)/specificity or 100 – 98/100) means that a woman with a negative test has 1 chance in 50 (or 2 in 100) of being pregnant (or 49 chances out of 50 of not being pregnant), and this –LR is then factored into the specific woman's pretest likelihood of being pregnant.

FALSE POSITIVE RATE AND FALSE NEGATIVE RATE

Two other test definitions less often used are false positive rate and false negative rate. For the pregnancy test **a false positive rate** is 0% (calculated as 100-specificity [100 – 100]). This is the proportion of women who received a positive test result when they were truly not pregnant.

The **false negative rate** is the proportion of women who received a negative test result when they are truly pregnant. For the pregnancy test, the false negative rate is 2% (calculated as 1-sensitivity or $100 - 98 = 2$).

Both false positive and false negative test results affect people's lives. With a false positive test result people assume incorrectly that they have the disease or condition they were tested for and become "labeled." People who think they are sick can actually start acting unwell even though they are healthy. They may miss time from work or refuse promotions and their general quality of life may deteriorate. This happened to men who worked in a steel mill after they were told incorrectly that they had high blood pressure.[3] False negative test results affect people's lives because individuals may not seek treatment when they should. For example, valuable treatment time is lost if the woman with breast cancer is told she does not have a malignancy when she really does.

One other way to describe this set of numbers is the number of false positive and the number of false negative patients in the group. The number of false positives is the number in the *b* box or cell of the 2×2 table and the number of false negatives is the number in the *c* box or cell of the 2×2 table; in our example these are 0 and 2, respectively.

RECEIVER OPERATING CHARACTERISTIC CURVES

Receiver Operating Characteristic Curves also called **Receiver Operator Characteristic (ROC)** curves are graphic representations of diagnostic test comparisons when the results can have ranges of values. Using cardiac enzyme levels to diagnose myocardial infarction, or various values for fasting blood glucose levels in persons who are suspected of having diabetes mellitus are examples where ROC curves can be useful. If the test has more than one possible cut point (laboratory value), or has a range of two or more test values, (for example, negative, weakly positive, and strongly positive) a ROC curve can be made plotting sensitivity and specificity on a graph. Each point on the graph, then, has its own sensitivity and specificity value. A "good" test will have a ROC value (area under the curve) of > 80%. Calculations are often done to find out what point or position on the curve (laboratory value) has the best combination of sensitivity and specificity.

It is essential for clinicians who make health care decisions using the above test characteristics to remember and work with the above nine definitions. For others, especially librarians who are using the terms for building search strategies, it is not as essential to learn the precise definitions of the terms. Most standard texts, including those listed in the appendix, have definitions if you need them. Remember that the most important aspects of diagnostic test results reporting are the sensitivity and specificity of the test. Next come the likelihood ratios for both positive and negative test results, the false positive rates and the false negative rates, and the predictive values. Predictive values, because of their changing values across populations, are currently less used than they once were. Likelihood ratios have become more important, and will increase in value over time.

UNDERSTANDING DIAGNOSTIC STATISTICS

Most clinicians do not routinely do their own calculations for diagnostic tests, but many find understanding the concepts easier if they complete a set of calculations. We will proceed using a clinical scenario of a 35-year-old woman who may have acute pancreatitis. Our diagnostic suspicion is high. Her symptoms include epigastric pain, anorexia, vomiting, nausea, and fever, and you know from previous encounters that she has a history of alcohol abuse.

Using data from a book of diagnostic strategies by Panzer and colleagues[4] to study a population of 200 persons with suspected pancreatitis, all would be given a new test, a serum lipase test. To evaluate whether the serum lipase test is a valid test (sensitivity and specificity over 80%), the results of the lipase test were compared with the diagnostic standard. An effective diagnostic standard for many diseases, including this one, is careful observation of the patient over time to determine whether the disease develops. The charts of all 200 persons were checked within 3 months, and each person was contacted by telephone to see if they had had pancreatitis. Both the chart reviewers and the telephone interviewers did not know the results of the lipase test for a given patient (blinding).

For the 200 persons tested, the chart audit and telephone contact showed that 53 had had pancreatitis and 147 did not. Of the 53 with pancreatitis, the lipase test was positive for 50 of the participants. Seven patients without pancreatitis had a positive lipase test. Fill in the following table (Table 3–2) and calculate the sensitivity and specificity, positive and negative likelihood ratios, positive and negative predictive values, and false positive and negative rates for the serum lipase test.

Table 3–2
2 × 2 Table for the Diagnosis of Pancreatitis

2 X 2 Table for Pancreatitis—Work Sheet

Disease/condition:_____ **(gold standard)**_____

	Positive +	Negative −	
New test + positive results	a	b	a + b
New test − negative results	c	d	c + d
	a + c	b + d	a + b + c + d

Sensitivity = a/(a + c)
= ___/(___+___)
= ___/___
= _____

Specificity = d/(b + d)
= ___/(___+___)
= ___/___

= _____

Positive Likelihood Ratio = sensitivity/(100 − specificity)
= _____/(100 − _____)
= _____/_____
= _____

Negative Likelihood Ratio = (100 − sensitivity)/specificity
= (100 − _____/(_____)
= _____/_____
= _____

Positive Predictive Value = a/(a + b)
= ___/(___+___)
= ___/___
= _____

Negative Predictive Value = d (c + d)
= ___/(___+___)
= ___/___
= _____

False Positive Rate = 100 − specificity
= 100 − (___)
= _____

False Negative Rate = 100 − specificity
= 100 − (___)
= _____

Table 3–2
2 × 2 Table for the Diagnosis of Pancreatitis continued

2 X 2 Table for Pancreatitis—Answers

	Disease/condition: Pancreatitis (gold standard) watchful waiting Positive +	Negative –	
New test: **serum lipase test** + positive results	50 a	7 b	57 a +b
New test: **serum lipase test** – negative results	c 3	d 140	c + d 143
	53 a + c	b + d	147 a + b + c + d 200

Sensitivity	= a/(a + c) = 50/(50 + 3) = 50/53 = **94% or 0.94**	**Specificity**	= d/(b + d) = 140/(7 + 140) = 140/147 = **95% or 0.95**
Positive Likelihood Ratio	= sens/(100 – spec) = 94/(100 – 95) = 94/5 = **18.8**	**Negative Likelihood Ratio**	= (100 – sens)/spec = (100 – 94)/95 = 6/95 = **0.06**
Positive Predictive Value	= a/(a + b) = 50/(50 + 7) = 50/57 = **88%**	**Negative Predictive Value**	= d (c + d) = 140 /(3 + 140) = 140/143 = **98%**
False Positive Rate	= 100 – specificity = 100 – 95 = **5%**	**False Negative Rate**	= 100 – sensitivity = 100 – 94 = **6%**

SUMMARY

In summary, diagnostic and screening test evaluations are done using a methodology that incorporates the following features. These features are in the order of importance that the Evidence-Based Medicine Working Group has designated in their User's Guide series.[5]

- The laboratory personnel who administer and evaluate or read the tests should be blinded to the results of the other tests being compared.
- The patient group should include persons with a spectrum of disease, from no disease to severe disease (often a large group of persons, not all of whom may have had the disease).

- A diagnostic or gold standard test already exists (for example, biopsy or a night in a sleep laboratory).
- Every person involved in the evaluation receives all the tests that are being evaluated. The order in which they receive the tests can be in random order, fixed order, or by convenience of the testing personnel or patients.
- Sets of test results are compared for being positive when the test result should be positive *and* negative when the test results should be negative.
- These agreements (that is, positive with positive and negative with negative) are measured using paired terms of sensitivity and specificity, positive and negative likelihood ratios, false and negative test rates, and positive and negative predictive values.

Indexers at NLM recognize most of the outcome measures (Table 3–3) but almost never index for the blinding or if the tests were done in random order. Comparative study is not a term that is used consistently by indexers. The CINAHL uses the terms sparingly as nurses often consider diagnosis to be broader and group the more "medical" terminology under terms such as assessment.

MEDLINE

MeSH, Subheadings, Publication Types, and Textwords for Diagnostic Studies

MeSH
Sensitivity and specificity*
    Predictive value of tests*
    ROC curves

Diagnostic errors
    False negative reactions
    False positive reactions
    Observer variation

Likelihood functions*
Diagnosis, differential*
Reproducibility of results
Area under curve
Probability

Subheadings
Diagnosis (for diagnosis of diseases and disorders)
    Radiography
    Radionuclide imaging
    Ultrasonography
Diagnostic use (for substances used in diagnosis)

Publication types
None

Textwords
Sensitivit:*
Specificit:*
Predictive value:
False positive
False negative
False rate:
Likelihood ratio:
Receiver operat: curve:
Pre test likelihood
Pretest likelihood
Post test likelihood
Posttest likehood
Post test probability
Posttest probability
ROC
Diagnostic standard:
Accurac: (combination of sensitivity and specificity)

Diagnosis, differential
The MeSH term "diagnosis, differential" is not a true diagnostic test research term. Instead, it is used to index an article that discusses two or more already established procedures to differentiate between similar diseases. You would use "diagnosis, differential" to retrieve citations that provide guidance for clinicians to be able to distinguish between Alzheimer's disease and depression in an elderly patient, or to distinguish between croup and whooping cough in a child.

---

*indicates a preferred term

CINAHL Database of Nursing and Allied Health Literature

CINAHL Index Terms and Subheadings for Diagnostic Studies

CINAHL Index Terms
Diagnosis
    Clinical assessment tools
    Diagnosis, differential
    Diagnosis, laboratory
        False negative reactions
        False positive reactions

Diagnostic errors
  Failure to diagnose
  False negative reactions
  False positive reactions
  Sensitivity and specificity
Validity
  Construct validity
    Sensitivity and specificity
    Predictive value of tests
  Measurement issues and assessments
    Reliability and validity
    Validity
      Construct validity
        Predictive value of tests
        Sensitivity and specificity

Observer bias
  Assimilator bias
  Central tendency bias
  Enhancement of contrast effect
  Error of leniency
  Error of severity
  Halo effect
  Reproducibility of results

Nursing assessment

CINAHL Subheadings
Diagnosis
Radiography
Ultrasonography
Diagnostic use
Nursing
Symptoms

CINAHL Document types
Nursing diagnoses
Practice guidelines
Systematic review
Research

PsycINFO

Descriptors, Publication Types, and Textwords for Diagnostic Studies

Descriptors
Diagnosis
   Computer Assisted Diagnosis
   Differential Diagnosis
   Educational Diagnosis
   Galvanic Skin Response

Medical Diagnosis+
   Biopsy
      Cardiography+
      Electrocardiography
   Dexamethasone Suppression Test

Echoencephalography

Electro Oculography

Electroencephalography+
   Alpha Rhythm
   Delta Rhythm
   Theta Rhythm

Electromyography

Electrostagmography

Electroplethysmography

Electroretinography

Encephalography+
   Echoencephalography
   Electroencephalography
      Alpha Rhythm
      Delta Rhythm
      Theta Rhythm
   Pneumoencephalography
   Rheoencephalography

Galvanic Skin Response

Ophthalmologic Examination+
   Electro Oculography
   Electroretinography

Plethysmography+
   Electroplethysmography

Pneumoencephalography

Prenatal Diagnsis

Rheoencephalography

Roentgenography+
   Angiography
   Mammography
   Pneumoencephalography

Tomography+
   Magnetic Resonance Imaging

Urinalysis
   Psychodiagnosis+
      Psychodiagnostic Interview+
         Diagnostic Interview Schedule

Differential Diagnosis

Screening

Ultrasound

Measurement+ (Definition: Conceptually broad array term referring to the process and tools used in psychological assessment of human subjects. Use specific test names or procedures if possible).

Testing+ (Definition: Administration of tests, and analysis and interpretation of test scores in order to measure differences between individuals or between test performances of the same individual on different occasions)

Testing Methods+

Methodology Descriptors

Predictive Validity+
Test Validity+
Statistical Validity+
Statistical Reliability+
Prediction Errors+
Maximum Likelihood
Predictability
Experimental Replication

Publication Type or Form/Content Type
Experimental Replication

Textwords
Sensitiv:*
Specific:*
ROC Curve:*
Diagnostic Error:*
False Positive:*
False Negative:*
Likelihood Ratio*
Accuracy

PsycINFO terms selected by Jean Sullivant

EMBASE/EXCERPTA MEDICA

Index Terms, Links, and EMTAGS for Diagnostic and Screening

Index terms
Diagnostic accuracy
Diagnostic error
Diagnostic value
Receiver operating characteristics
Differential diagnosis
Area under the curve

Links (subheadings)
Diagnosis

Emtags (publication types)
Diagnosis

MEDLINE HEDGES

The hedges described in the therapy chapter were developed and evaluated as MEDLINE search strategies that retrieve only the ready-for-clinical-application studies we are discussing.[6] They were evaluated using the diagnostic test evaluation process, and were developed to retrieve all possible relevant citations based on research methodology (for example, randomized controlled trials for treatment or prevention issues); and at the same time to not retrieve, or retrieve the minimum number of, citations of articles of lesser quality. In other words, we wanted a search that was positive as often as it should be positive, and negative when it should have been negative: we wanted our search strategies to retrieve the relevant citations as often as possible (high sensitivity), and not retrieve the less-relevant citations as often as possible (high specificity).

For the Hedges Project, as we called it, the "disease" or "condition" we studied was a set of methodologically sound citations. The setting was the MEDLINE database. The gold standard we used in the research process was carefully defined. Three readers, under the supervision of the principal investigator of the study, read and classified articles into categories of research and then according to whether each article passed methodologic criteria. Reading was done in triplicate until the readers were able to complete the assessments with 90% perfect agreement. Once this inter-rater reliability check was done, each reader continued reading until all 10 journals were read for 1986 and 1991.

The new test was a series of search strategies suggested by librarians, clinician searchers, and NLM staff. These terms, phrases, and index terms were used to retrieve citations which were then used to evaluate the effectiveness of the NLM indexing. Measures of sensitivity (what proportion of the available relevant articles in the 10 journals were retrieved) and specificity (what proportion of the irrelevant articles in the 10 journals did the search strategy *not* retrieve) were calculated for each term individually and in combination with other terms. In standard search terminology, all eight measures of diagnostic test evaluation characteristics were determined for each search item. For retrieving the most (largest number of) relevant citations, the best single term in MEDLINE is **sensitivity (textword)**. The diagnostic strategy with the highest sensitivity (most relevant articles with the least [smallest number of] irrelevant articles) is:

> **explode sensitivity a#d specificity (MeSH)**
> **OR all sensitivity (textword)**
> **OR diagnosis (pre-exploded subheading)**
> **OR diagnostic use (subheading)**
> **OR specificity (textword)**

The diagnostic strategy with the highest specificity (most relevant articles possible) is:

> **explode sensitivity a#d specificity (mesh)**
> **OR predictive value: (textword)**

Example 3–1
Baxt WG, Skora J. Prospective validation of artificial neural network trained to identify acute myocardial infarction. Lancet 1996;347:12–5.

This study evaluated 1070 patients with chest pain who came to the emergency department of a hospital in California. The study compared the performance of residents and attending staff in discerning which patients were having a myocardial infarction with the performance of a computer system using the data collected by the same physicians. The data included information from the history, physical examination, and the electrocardiogram. The diagnostic standard was careful watching of the patients over time, coupled with a chart audit and patient contact. Sensitivity and specificity and likelihood ratios were calculated for the physicians, and the computer program that used the physician-collected data.

Outcomes of the study were that 818 adults had noncardiac chest pain, 102 had angina, 75 had unstable angina, and 75 had a myocardial infarction. The physicians' assess-

MEDLINE Record for Example 3–1

Unique Identifier 96129893

Authors Baxt WG. Skora J.

Institution Department of Emergency Medicine, University of California, San Diego, Medical Center, USA.

Title Prospective validation of artificial neural network trained to identify acute myocardial infarction [see comments].

Source Lancet. 347(8993):12–5, 1996 Jan 6.

MeSH Subject Headings

Chest Pain/di [Diagnosis]	Male
Comparative Study	Middle Age
Electrocardiography	*Myocardial Infarction/di [Diagnosis]
Emergency Medicine	*Neural Networks (Computer)
Emergency Service, Hospital	Physicians
Female	Prospective Studies
Follow-Up Studies	Reproducibility of Results
Human	Sensitivity and Specificity

Abstract
BACKGROUND: Artificial neural networks apply nonlinear statistics to pattern recognition problems. One such problem is acute myocardial infarction (AMI), a diagnosis which, in a patient presenting as an emergency, can be difficult to confirm. We report here a prospective comparison of the **diagnostic accuracy** of a network and that of physicians, on the same patients with suspected AMI. METHODS: Emergency department physicians who evaluated 1070 patients 18 years or older presenting to the emergency department of a teaching hospital in California, USA with anterior chest pain indicated whether they thought these patients had sustained a myocardial infarction. The network analyzed the patient data collected by the physicians during their evaluations and also generated a diagnosis. FINDINGS: The physicians had a diagnostic **sensitivity** and **specificity** for myocardial infarction of 73.3% (95% confidence interval 63.3–83.3%) and 81.1% (78.7–83.5%), respectively, while the network had a diagnostic sensitivity and specificity of 96.0% (91.2–100%) and 96.0% (94.8–97.2%), respectively. Only 7% of patients had had an AMI, a low frequency but typical for anterior chest pain. INTERPRETATION: The application of nonlinear neural computational analysis via an artificial neural network to the clinical diagnosis of myocardial infarction appears to have significant potential.

Publication Type Journal Article.

ments for determining a myocardial infarction had a sensitivity and specificity of 73% and 81%, and positive and negative likelihood ratios of 3.9 and 0.3, respectively. The computer program, after it had "learned" on a series of patients, had a sensitivity and specificity of 96% and 96%, and positive and negative likelihood ratios of 24 and 0.04, respectively. The outcomes of this study suggest that computers may play an important role in helping physicians become better diagnosticians in certain situations and settings.

Retrieval Strategy Can Use Any of the Following:

MeSH indexing	Comparative study
	Reproducibility of results
	Sensitivity and specificity
Textwords	Diagnostic accuracy (abstract)
	Sensitivity (abstract)
	Specificity (abstract)

Example 3–2
Cutler AF, Havstad S, Ma CK, Blaser MJ, Perez-Perez GI, Schubert TT. Accuracy of invasive and noninvasive tests to diagnose *Helicobacter pylori* infection. Gastroenterology 1995;109:136–41.

This study assessed the various diagnostic and screening tests for *Helicobacter pylori* infection. Six diagnostic tests (7 sets of test results) were compared. Three were invasive, involving endoscopies, and three were noninvasive blood or breath tests. No gold standard exists for detection of *H. pylori* infection, and therefore a diagnostic standard was set by the investigators using a concordance of four of the seven test results as the gold standard—if four of the test results agree this is "truth."

Two hundred and sixty-eight patients received all six tests. Eighty-two patients had duodenal ulcers, 49 had gastric ulcers, eight had pylori channel ulcers, 55 had nonulcer dyspepsia, and 65% were considered to have *H. pylori* infection using the concordance rule of four or more test results being in agreement. All tests performed well with a blood-based test and a breath test performing as well as a test using endoscopic biopsy techniques. Currently many medical centers use the breath tests for determining *H.pylori* infection status.

Retrieval Strategy Can Use Any of the Following:

MeSH indexing	Predictive value of tests
	Sensitivity and specificity
	Comparative study
Textwords	Diagnose (title and abstract)
	Sensitivity (abstract)
	Specificity (abstract)
	Negative and positive predictive value (abstract)
	Accurat: (abstract)

MEDLINE Record for Example 3–2

Unique Identifier 95317532

Authors Cutler AF. Havstad S. Ma CK. Blaser MJ. Perez-Perez GI. Schubert TT.

Institution Division of Gastroenterology, Henry Ford Hospital, Detroit, Michigan, USA.

Title **Accuracy** of invasive and noninvasive tests to **diagnose** *Helicobacter pylori* infection [see comments].

Source Gastroenterology. 109(1):136–41, 1995 Jul.

MeSH Subject Headings

Adult	Human
Aged	IgA/bl [Blood]
Aged, 80 and over	IgG/bl [Blood]
Biopsy	Logistic Models
Breath Tests	Male
Chi-Square Distribution	Middle Age
Comparative Study	**Predictive Value of Tests**
Female	Pyloric Antrum/pa [Pathology]
Helicobacter pylori/im [Immunology]	**Sensitivity and Specificity**
*Helicobacter pylori	Staining
*Helicobacter Infections/di [Diagnosis]	Urea/an [Analysis]
Helicobacter Infections/im [Immunology]	

Abstract

BACKGROUND & AIMS: Multiple tests are available for determining *Helicobacter pylori* infection. Our aim was to compare the **sensitivity, specificity,** and **negative and positive predictive value** of the most widely available tests for diagnosis of H. pylori. METHODS: A total of 268 patients (mean age, 53.7 ± 15.8 years; 142 male and 126 female; 125 white and 143 nonwhite) was tested for *H. pylori* infection by [13C]urea breath test (UBT), measurement of serum immunoglobulin (Ig) G and IgA antibody levels, and antral biopsy specimens for CLO test, histology, and Warthin-Starry stain. No patient received specific treatment for *H. pylori* before testing. The infection status for each patient was established by a concordance of test results. RESULTS: Warthin-Starry staining had the best sensitivity and specificity, although CLO test, UBT, and IgG levels were not statistically different in determining the correct diagnosis. The absence of chronic antral inflammation was the best method to exclude infection. Stratification of results by clinical characteristics showed that UBT and chronic inflammation were the best predictors of *H. pylori* status in patients older than 60 years of age. IgA was a better predictor in white patients. CONCLUSIONS: The noninvasive UBT and IgG serology test are as **accurate** in predicting *H. pylori* status in untreated patients as the invasive tests of CLO and Warthin-Starry.

Publication Type Clinical Trial. Journal Article.

Example 3–3

Offenbacher H, Fazekas F, Schmidt R, et al. Assessment of MRI criteria for a diagnosis of MS. Neurology 1993;43:905–9.

Multiple sclerosis is a disease that had traditionally been hard to diagnose. This study was done to assess various criteria from the magnetic resonance imaging (MRI) readings to best balance the sensitivity and specificity results for diagnosing multiple sclerosis. It involved reading the MRI scans from 1528 consecutive patients. Blinded chart review was the diagnostic standard. Sensitivities and specificities varied with the sensitivities often being higher. High sensitivities are useful for "ruling out" a disease and high specificities are useful for "ruling in" a disease. Because the sensitivities here are high, MRI studies are useful for telling patients with symptoms that they do not have multiple sclerosis if they have a negative test result.

Retrieval Strategies Can Use Any of the Following:

MeSH indexing	Comparative study
	Predictive value of tests
	Sensitivity and specificity
Textwords	Diagnosis (title and abstract)
	Sensitivity (abstract)
	Specificity (abstract)
	Positive predictive value (abstract)
	Unaware of patients (abstract)

ASSIGNMENT

Note that physicians and mental health professionals are more interested than nurses in screening or diagnostic questions. Try these searches in MEDLINE and, if you think appropriate, in PsycINFO.

1. A small bowel biopsy is invasive, especially in children. The gliadin antibody test is a blood-based test. How accurate (combined sensitivity and specificity) is the test for diagnosing celiac disease? Has it ever been used for screening purposes?

2. D-dimer levels (again, a blood-based test) show promise for detecting deep venous thrombosis (DVT) for stroke patients who sometimes cannot verbalize pain in their legs. Painful legs in recently immobilized patients are often a good indication that DVT could be present. What is the sensitivity and specificity of the D-dimer test? For all DVT? For proximal (between the knee and hip) DVT?

3. Multiple sclerosis is a long-term, progressive neurological disease that has traditionally been difficult to diagnosis. Multiple sclerosis was said to be present if many other diseases such as brain tumors and pernicious anemia were excluded (ruled out). What tests are now routine for patients with signs and symptoms of multiple sclerosis? What is the usual gold standard in the diagnosis of multiple sclerosis?

MEDLINE Record for Example 3–3

Unique Identifier   93261610

Authors   Offenbacher H. Fazekas F. Schmidt R. Freidl W. Flooh E. Payer F. Lechner H.

Institution   Department of Neurology, Karl-Franzens University, Graz, Austria.

Title   Assessment of MRI criteria for a **diagnosis** of MS.

Source   Neurology. 43(5):905–9, 1993 May.

MeSH Subject Headings

Adolescence	Magnetic Resonance Imaging/mt [Methods]
Adult	*Magnetic Resonance Imaging
Aged	Male
Aged, 80 and over	Middle Age
*Brain/pa [Pathology]	*Multiple Sclerosis/di [Diagnosis]
Comparative Study	Multiple Sclerosis/pa [Pathology]
Female	**Predictive Value of Tests**
Human	**Sensitivity and Specificity**

Abstract
To test the reliability of four previously proposed MRI criteria for the diagnosis of MS, we reviewed 1,500 consecutive brain scans for the presence, number, size, and location of areas of increased signal (AIS) on proton-density and T2-weighted images, **unaware of the patients'** clinical presentations and ages. This series included 134 subjects with a clinical diagnosis of MS. Relying exclusively on the presence of at least three or four AIS for a positive diagnosis of MS resulted in high **sensitivity** (90% for three AIS and 87% for four) but inadequate **specificity** (71% for three AIS and 74% for four) and **positive predictive value** (23% for three AIS and 25% for four). If one of these lesions was required to border the lateral ventricles, specificity was 92% and positive predictive value was 50% at a sensitivity of 87%. Using the Fazekas criteria (at least three AIS and two of the following features: abutting body of lateral ventricles, infratentorial lesion location, and size > 5 mm) led to a further highly significant improvement of specificity (96%; p = 0.0000) and increase of the positive predictive value (65%) at the expense of a less significant decrease in sensitivity (81%; p < 0.01).

Publication Type   Journal Article.

---

4. If you slip and fall on the ice in eastern Ontario you might not get an automatic x-ray in the emergency department to ascertain if a bone in the ankle area is broken or needs further evaluation. Does a good clinical (hands-on) test exist to assess the likelihood of fracture among patients with ankle pain that can be used by primary care health workers?

5. Can short questionnaires be used for screening for depression in routine or primary care settings?

REFERENCES

1. Irwin K, Olivo N, Schable CA, et al, and the CDC-Bronx-Lebanon HIV Serosurvey Team. Performance characteristics of a rapid HIV antibody assay in a hospital with a high prevalence of HIV infection. Ann Intern Med 1996;125:471–5.

2. Sackett DL, Straus S. On some clinically useful measures of the accuracy of diagnostic testing. ACP J Club 1998 Sep–Oct;129:A17–9.

3. Johnston ME, Gibson ES, Terry CW, et al. Effects of labelling on income, work and social function among hypertensive employees. J Chronic Dis 1984;37:417–23.

4. Panzer RJ, Black ER, Griner PF, editors. Diagnostic strategies for common medical problems. Philadelphia (PA): American College of Physicians; 1991. p. 160.

5. Jaeschke R, Guyatt GH, Sackett DL for the Evidence-Based Medicine Working Group. Users' guides to the medical literature. III. How to use an article about a diagnostic test. A. Are the results of the study valid? JAMA 1994;271:389–91.

6. Haynes RB, Wilczynski NL, McKibbon KA, et al. Developing optimal search strategies for detecting clinically sound studies in MEDLINE. J Am Med Inform Assoc 1994;1:447–58.

4

Etiology, Causation, and Harm

Another very important area of health care research is **etiology** or **causation**. An alternative word for it is **harm**. This term is used when clinicians refer to drug studies and their adverse effects. Assessment of etiology, causation, or harm is becoming more important as people become aware of the choices they have in relation to prevention and control of diseases and conditions. Often topics of interest for etiology and causation are long-term issues, such as the effects of exercise during adulthood decreasing the risk for osteoporosis in women after menopause, or whether exposure to electromagnetic energy fields from electric power lines causes leukemia in children.

FOUR METHODOLOGIES FOR EVALUATING ETIOLOGY

Briefly, an evaluation of a causation topic assesses exposures or risk factors and the related disease outcomes. For example, does having dental fillings that contain mercury, owning pets early in life, living in cooler climates, having had optic neuritis, or being a woman increase one's risk for developing multiple sclerosis? At various times, researchers have felt that all of these factors might be related to an increased risk for multiple sclerosis. Conversely, the following factors have been considered to be "protective" or to reduce the risk for development of multiple sclerosis: no pets during childhood, no dental caries, living in tropical climates, not having had optic neuritis, or being a man. For the purposes of this book we will assume that etiology refers to both the increased risk for development and protection against a disease or condition. Not all researchers, however, agree with both the increased risk and protective factors being called "causation." Indexers who produce MEDLINE and other databases separate the two into distinct categories: they consider the increased risk to be "etiology" and the protective effects to be "prevention and control."

Etiology research can be done using at least four different methodologies. Their quality, time point when the exposures and outcomes are assessed, and relative frequency of publication are shown below in Table 4–1. The four methods vary in many aspects—most importantly, in quality (strength of evidence) and frequency of publication. Generally, studies with the highest methodologic quality are considered at the narrowest part of the wedge: the most appropriate for clinical decision-making.

Table 4–1
Study Designs Used in Etiology Research

Type	Quality Rating	Time of Exposure	Frequency of Publication
Randomized controlled trials	*****	Future	*
Cohort studies	***	Present	**
Case-control studies	*	Past	***
Cross sectional studies with statistically adjusted groups	—	?	*****

Clinical Example: Birds and Lung Cancer

Because of the four ways to assess it, etiology is probably one of the most complex, if not the most difficult, of the categories to understand and apply. The best way to start is with a concrete clinical example and work with it referring to the features listed in Table 4–1.

In the late 1980s, Dutch researchers noticed that people with lung cancer quite often had pet birds.[1] Several other lung diseases, such as bird fancier's lung, are associated with keeping pet birds or raising fowl, so this hypothesis may have some biologic rationale. To test their hypothesis that the pet birds caused lung cancer, the researchers could have used any of the four methodologies from the table above.

Randomized Controlled Trials

Using the strongest methodology, the **randomized controlled trial**, they would have assembled a group of people and randomly allocated them to have or not to have pet birds. After many years the researchers would assess the people in both groups to see whether they had developed lung cancer. As for therapy studies, the rates of lung cancer in each group would be compared and conclusions drawn from the data. This study is probably ethically possible, but not very practical or fundable. The question of birds and lung cancer, as with many other etiology research questions, must be answered using research designs other than the randomized controlled trial.

Cohort Studies

The next strongest methodology for testing etiology questions is the **cohort study**. The term *cohort* comes from the Latin word for "group": a cohort was the smallest unit of a Roman army, equivalent to 10 men. Cohort studies follow a group of people over time and measure outcomes. Researchers gather people who do not have the outcome of interest, such as recurrent otitis media in preschool children. They then ascertain which children in the cohort or group have been exposed to the possible causative agent: in this case, secondhand tobacco smoke exposure (having parents and other adult members of the households who smoke). After a period of time, the research staff compares the number of children in each group (the group with exposure to secondhand smoke and the group without exposure) that have developed the disease in question (ear infections).

A cohort study of the question of caged birds increasing the risk for lung cancer would start with some people who have pet birds and some people who do not have them. The research staff would compare the bird owners with persons who had similar baseline characteristics, but who did not keep pet birds, to assess all participants for a period of time to find out how many bird owners and nonbird owners developed cancer. The study would probably take many years to complete, because as with most exposures, the time between exposure to birds and outcomes is often a long one. The comparison with a control group is crucial for the accuracy of the results. The confounders in the study must be assessed and factored into the final analysis. **Confounders** are the factors, other than the one being studied, that could account for naturally-occurring differences between the groups. For this study, the confounding factors are such things as smoking, living next to or downwind from large industrial sites, or a strong family history of breast cancer. Measurement of these confounding factors at baseline, during the study, and at the end of the study can then be factored into the analysis, and their effects are considered to "cancel out" or are adjusted for in the presentation of the final results. The analysis that takes into account or specifically analyzes for the differences among the groups is called **multivariate analysis** or **multiple regression analysis**. At study end, researchers want to assess the effect of having birds as pets while taking into account other potential confounding factors. (All research, including randomized controlled trials, must also consider the issues of confounders and bias. The randomization process is designed to balance the rates of various confounders in each group. Therefore confounders, although an important issue in randomized, controlled trials, are not as important as in the other methods of assessing causation.) Bias is the often unintentional tendency to assess or measure things not as they are but as what one thinks they should be. For example the detection bias occurs when we think we should be finding "something" and we continue to look for it even if it isn't there. If one continues to test children for giftedness, more and more will be children identified. Biases cannot be as easily factored into analyses as confounders are; therefore researchers must work hard to recognize and eliminate bias before it occurs. Jadad[2] summarizes bias very well in his book on clinical trials.

The results of cohort studies, as for randomized controlled trial studies of etiology questions, are presented as **relative risks** (**RR**) with confidence intervals: a statistical approximation of the increased risk for the outcome that the exposure studied conferred on the study participants. (See the end of this section for a fuller definition and an example of a calculation of relative risk.) Relative risk is the measure of the risk involved if you have the exposure (birds) that you will develop the outcome (lung cancer).

Case-Control Studies

The **case-control study** is a less powerful methodology than the randomized controlled trial and the cohort study. It goes back in time to assess exposure for the people who are being evaluated. Researchers take persons with the disease or other outcome of interest (lung cancer, in the pet bird example) and match each person with cancer with another person who does not have it but who is similar in other features or confounding factors. For each member of these pairs, the researchers check back in time for the presence or absence of the causative agent. In our example, the investigators would pair each patient with lung cancer with another person of similar age, smoking habits, living conditions, and so on who does not have that disease. They would then count how many men and women in each group had owned pet birds. If more people with lung cancer had pet birds, one would conclude that an association may exist between them. The results of case-control studies are presented as **odds ratios (OR)**. (See the end of this section for definition and calculation.) The odds ratio is a measure of the likelihood you were exposed to the risk factor (birds) now that you have the outcome (lung cancer).

The case-control study design is considered "weak," or at least weaker than some designs, because exposure data are usually collected by asking people to remember and report on exposures that happened many years before. Often the best thing that can be said about human memory is that it is selective. An example of where reporting of previous exposures can be biased is in the question of whether breastfeeding (exposure) is protective against breast cancer (the disease outcome). In a case-control study, women with breast cancer may remember and report their history of breastfeeding differently than women who do not have it. Another example of where remembering exposures can be problematic is a study of the long-term consequences of using aluminum pots and pans for everyday cooking. Some research shows that aluminum exposure increases the risk for development of Alzheimer's disease. In a case-control study, asking men and women with Alzheimer's disease to report on the constitution of their pots and pans over the past 50 to 60 years might not be the best way to collect data to answer the question.

Cross-Sectional Studies with Statistically Adjusted Groups

Cross-sectional studies that use statistical adjustment of groups can also be used to compare one group of persons with another and make deductions about cause and effect. Many truths have first been recognized using this kind of research; many misrepresentations have also occurred. Examples are numerous in the literature for both. Using cross-sectional studies to answer our question about birds and lung cancer, the researchers would have taken a group of persons with lung cancer and another group of persons without it and compared the bird-keeping rates. Groups are often convenience samples obtained from shopping malls, workplaces, nursing homes, universities, or other locations. Researchers rely on statisticians to adjust the findings from the groups to correct or balance for confounders and problems associated with the cross-sectional research methodology. The biggest methodology problem associated with cross-sectional studies is that both the exposure and the outcomes are assessed at the same time, and no one can tell which came first. For example, a cross-sectional study would not be able to assess if depression caused men to be overweight or being overweight caused men to be depressed: the cross-sectional study could only measure the rates of being depressed and being overweight in a group of people.

Horst et al., the Dutch researchers who first postulated the association between birds and lung cancer, completed a case-control study and found a positive association between pet birds and lung cancer[1]—more persons with lung cancer than without had kept birds. Because their study was a case-control study, and thus not a strong design, the question has not completely been answered, and people have not been told to stop keeping birds because of fears of lung cancer. Research with stronger methods must be done before this question can be fully answered.

Comparison of Designs

In summary, the cross-sectional studies with statistically adjusted groups are the easiest to complete, and are a fast way to do etiology research. Most clinicians, however, do not consider such studies to be valid enough to use in forming health care decisions, especially if studies with stronger methodology exist. These cross-sectional studies are often used for an initial, quick check on an idea, (for example, does an association exist between aluminum cooking pots and Alzheimer's disease?). Case-control studies are marginally harder to do, and may take a little more time than cross-sectional studies with statistically adjusted groups, but they have methodology that is somewhat stronger.

Even though case-control studies are considered to have relatively weak methodology, they have a place in health care research. They can be used to study rare side effects of treatments, because researchers do not need to assemble a large number of study participants. Case-control studies can be done relatively quickly, because the researchers do not have to wait until the disease or condition develops: the disease is already present, and only the exposures from the past need to be assessed. Doll and Hill used a case-control study to be among the first to show an association between tobacco smoking and lung cancer.[3] The associations between toxic shock syndrome and tampon use[4] and between Reye's syndrome and aspirin use in children[5] were both shown in well-done case-control studies. Because the studies could be done quickly once researchers came to suspect the associations, lives were saved and suffering alleviated.

Cohort studies are harder to do, and take even more time to complete, than case-control studies: in cohort studies the disease or other outcomes will develop in the future. Cohort studies have a stronger methodology, and therefore their evidence is considered stronger than that of case-control studies when making clinical decisions. Randomized controlled trials have both the strongest methodology and the strongest evidence, but they are difficult, if not impossible, to do to answer etiology questions.

ISSUES

Ethics

Ethics are important in studies of etiology. Researchers cannot control each person's exposures or risk factors for diseases and conditions. These exposures or risk factors can be "good" or protective (for example, advanced education or no family history of diabetes mellitus), or "bad" or associated with an increased risk (for example, high blood pressure or age ≥ 85 years). Logistics play a role similar to that of ethics because of the difficulty of controlling exposures, such as living next to factories or electric lines and the length of time it takes for a disease or condition to develop. For example, some endocrinologists feel that early exposure to cow's milk is a risk factor for developing diabetes mellitus in later life. To assess this, a randomized controlled trial is probably not feasible, because few mothers would consent to being randomized to either breastfeed their children or use cow's milk for their newborn infants. Some research shows that cow's milk is not good for infants less than a year old because of allergy, nutritional, and other problems. A cohort design presents similar problems. In addition, children would have to be followed for at least 20 years to be able to assess the rates of development of adult-onset diabetes. A case-control study or one with a cross-sectional design with statistically adjusted groups may be the only possible alternative to evaluate the question of an association between cow's milk exposure and the development of diabetes mellitus during adulthood.

Blinding

From a methodological point of view, blinding is probably the most important issue in causation studies. It is slightly more important for the studies with weaker methodologies: case-control studies and cross-sectional studies with statistically adjusted groups. All study designs must assess both exposures and outcomes, but this assessment is done at different times for each of the four study types. Exposure is assessed in the future for randomized controlled trials, in the present for cohort studies, and in the past for case-control studies and cross-sectional studies with statistically adjusted groups. The people who assess the exposures (for example, high I.Q.) must be blinded to the outcomes (for example, high income at age 40) *and* the persons who assess the outcomes (for example, high income at age 40) must be blinded to the exposures (for example, high I.Q.). Blinding is less important when the outcomes are objective. This means that if the outcome for an etiology study is all-cause mortality, the blinding is not as important—a death is a death, is a death... Other examples of objective outcomes are confirmed divorces, birthweight, or a laboratory confirmed diagnosis when the laboratory-output is taken from a machine and involves little chance for misreading the results. Even though blinding is crucial for these studies, it is not indexed by MEDLINE.

Association Versus Causation

Another important issue in understanding etiology is that, just because two things occur at the same time (are associated), one does not necessarily cause the other. As a rather extreme example, the rate of influenza is lower in the summer than in the winter. People also eat more ice cream in the summer. No one would, however, link eating ice cream with a decreased risk for the flu. Health care personnel regularly struggle with the issue of association not being the same as causation. One example of this is a series of ongoing Finnish studies by Salonen et al.[6] In 1992 they reported that persons who had a myocardial infarction also had high levels of stored iron in their blood. The only effective, low-cost clinical method of reducing iron levels is bloodletting. Some blood donor organizations, using this association data, have developed an advertising program that encourages persons to donate blood to reduce their risk for having a myocardial infarction. Not all researchers or clinicians believe that the iron levels-and-heart attack association is true. They feel that the association found by Salonen et al. has not been proved with sufficient strength of evidence that such decisions as the development and use of aggressive advertising programs to increase blood donor response are justified. Etiology studies must be assessed carefully, and common sense must be applied in understanding and using them for clinical decisions.

HOW RESULTS OF ETIOLOGY STUDIES ARE REPORTED

Relative Risk

Both relative risks (RR) and odds ratios (OR) are used to statistically represent the associations found in etiology studies. **Relative risk** is the risk or rate of developing a disease in the exposed group divided by the risk or rate of developing the disease in those who were not exposed. Cohort studies and randomized controlled trials present their findings using RR.

An example of using RR to present data comes from the Nurses' Health Study.[7] Willet et al. found that women who had gained at least 20 to 25 pounds since they were 18 years old had a lifetime RR for developing coronary heart disease of 1.9. This means that women who had gained 20 to 25 or more pounds had 1.9 more times the risk for developing coronary heart disease than women who had gained little or no weight beyond their teenage weight: basically, double the rate. Using hypothetical data we can see how this RR of 1.9 was calculated.

Of 200 women with a weight gain of at least 20 to 25 pounds, 106 women developed coronary heart disease during their lifetime. This risk or rate is calculated using the data: 106/200, which is 53%. In 200 women with long-term stable weight, only 58 developed coronary heart disease. This risk or rate is calculated as 58/200, or 26%. To calculate the RR, we take these two risks and form a ratio: the rate in women with exposure divided by the rate in women without exposure. The calculation for the RR is thus 53%/26%, or 1.9.

Odds Ratio

Odds ratios (OR) are used to report findings from case-control studies. An OR is the ratio of the rate among people who have a disease of having been exposed in the past to the rate of exposure in the past among people who do not have the disease. For example, DiFranza et al.[8] report that children who were hospitalized for lower respiratory infections have an OR of 3.3 for being exposed to parental tobacco smoke. This means that children who were hospitalized with lower respiratory infection were 3.3 times more likely to have been exposed to parental tobacco smoke than their peers who were hospitalized with a condition other than lower respiratory infections.

SUMMARY

The Evidence-Based Working Group, in their Users' Guide,[9] lists the aspects of etiology methods in the following order of clinical importance.

- similarity of clearly identified comparison groups with respect to important determinants of outcome, other than the one of interest (confounders).
- outcomes and exposures measurements done in the same way in the groups being compared.
- follow-up of sufficient length.

Secondary determinants of strength include

- assessment of a temporal relationship (for example, did people smoke before they got lung cancer?)
- a dose-response gradient (for example, did heavier smokers get lung cancer sooner or at a higher rate, was the disease more severe?)
- the strength of the association between exposure and outcome
- the precision of the estimate of risk.

Indexers often recognize the study methodology for randomized controlled trials, cohort studies, case-control studies, and cross-sectional studies with statistically adjusted groups. In addition they index for risk in various forms and OR. Indexers, however, use risk only for the increase in probability of the disease or condition (for example, a family history of colorectal cancer increases one's risk for colorectal cancer). For the "protective" effects (for example, hormone replacement therapy reduces the risk for Alzheimer's disease) the indexers use subheadings and indexing related to prevention and control. Possible indexing terms and phrases for all four databases are on the following pages.

MEDLINE

Mesh, Subheadings, and Textwords for Etiology and Causation Studies

MeSH
Study characteristics (non-MeSH)
    Analytic studies

Case-control studies*
　　Retrospective studies (means back in time)
Cohort studies*
　　Longitudinal studies
　　　　Prospective studies (means forward in time)
　　　　Follow-up studies
Cross-sectional studies
Risk*
Risk assessment
　　Risk factors
Odds ratio
Causality
Logistic models
Epidemiologic factors
　　Age factors
　　Comorbidity
　　Precipitation factors
Risk assessment

Subheadings
Etiology
Prevention and control
Adverse effects
Poisoning
Epidemiology (for distributions, causes, and attributes of disease)
Toxicity
Genetic
Chemically induced

Textwords
Cohort
Case control:
Case comparison
Case referent
Risk
Relative risk
Causation or causal:
Odds ratio:
Etiol: or aetiol:

---

*indicates a preferred term

CINAHL Database of Nursing and Allied Health Literature

CINAHL Index Terms and Subheadings for Etiology and Causation Studies

CINAHL Index terms
Analytic research
Risk factors
    Cardiovascular risk factors
Risk assessment
Odds ratio
Non-experimental studies
    Case control studies
        Hospital-based case control
        Matched case control
        Population-based case control
    Correlational studies
    Prospective studies

Prospective studies
    Concurrent prospective studies
    Nonconcurrent prospective studies
    Panel studies
        Retrospective panel studies
        Revolving panel studies
    Pseudolongitudinal studies

Professional practice, research based
    Nursing practice, research based

Epidemiological research
    Seroprevalence studies

Subheadings
Etiology
Prevention and control
Adverse effects
Poisoning
Epidemiology
Familial and genetic
Nursing (also gets lots of therapy and diagnosis studies)
Chemically induced

Document types
Research

Textwords
Use MEDLINE terms above

CINAHL thesaurus terms provided by Katy Nesbit
All extracts from the CINAHL® Thesaurus Copyright © 1999, Cinahl Information Systems. Reprinted with permission from Cinahl Information Systems.

PsycINFO

Descriptors, Publication Types, and Textwords for Etiology and Causation

Descriptors
At Risk Populations
Coronary Prone Behavior
Predisposition
Susceptability (Disorders)
Etiology
Ethnospecific Disorders+
Attribution
Prevention+
Side Effects (Drug)+
Toxicity
Epidemiology

Methodology Descriptors
Between Groups Design
Cohort Analysis
Follow-up Studies
Longitudinal Studies
Repeated Measures
Empirical Methods+
Experimental Methods
Observation Methods
Causal Analysis
Cohort Analysis

Experimental Subjects
    Experiment Volunteers

Experiment Controls (Used for Control groups)

Publication Type or Form/ Content Type
Empirical Study
Follow-up Study

Longitudinal Study
Prospective Study
Retrospective Study

Keywords
Risk
Odds ratio
Cohort
Case control
Relative risk
Causation or causal:*
Etiol:* or aetiol:*
Analytic stud:*
Cross sectional stud:*
Harm

PsycINFO terms selected by Jean Sullivant

EMBASE/EXCERPTA MEDICA

Index Terms, Links, and EMTAGS for Etiology and Causation Studies

Index terms
Case control study
Longitudinal study
Prospective study
Retrospective study
Cohort analysis
Risk
 Cardiovascular risk
 Explosive risk
 Genetic risk
 High risk patient
 High risk population
 High risk pregnancy
 Infection risk
 Population risk
 Recurrence risk
 Risk assessment
 Risk benefit analysis
 Risk factor
 Risk management

Links (subheadings)
Adverse drug reactions
Drug interaction
Drug toxicity
Complication
Congenital disorder
Etiology
Heredity
Side effect

Emtags (publication types)
Adverse drug reactions
Etiology
Fatality
Iatrogenic disease
Intoxication
Congenital disorder

MEDLINE HEDGES

MEDLINE hedges have been done for etiology studies. The best single term is:

risk (textword)

The hedge with the highest sensitivity (most relevant citations combined with fewest irrelevant citations) is:

explode cohort studies (MeSH)
OR exp risk (MeSH)
OR odds ratio: (textword)
OR relative risk (textword)
OR case control: (textword)

The MEDLINE with the highest specificity search strategy (the most relevant citations possible) is:

case-control studies (MeSH)
OR cohort (textword)

Example 4–1
Randomized controlled trial
Kay D, Fleisher JM, Salmon RL, et al. Predicting likelihood of gastroenteritis from sea bathing: results from randomised exposure. Lancet 1994;344:905–9.

This study is a randomized controlled trial assessing whether sea bathing in the U. K. is associated with an increase in gastroenteritis. It is one of the few randomized controlled trials in the etiology and causation category. It concludes that sea bathing is not good for your stomach's health, but some of the features of it make one wonder if the funding for this study might have been better spent on other projects. Some of these features are based on common sense, and include:

- How common is sea bathing in Britain?
- Can the results of a British study of British beaches be used in other areas of the world?
- How realistic or reasonable are the study conditions and results (see below)? The conditions of the study seem artificial and contrived.

The study took four summers to complete, and was done at four U.K. sea resorts. One thousand two hundred and sixteen adults agreed to participate, and after signing consent letters came to the beach ready for swimming. Once on the beach each person was examined by a physician, and then half were randomly allocated to bathe in a defined, roped-off 20-meter area of the sea for at least 10 minutes. They had to completely immerse their heads at least three times, and their location and duration of exposure were closely monitored by study staff located on the beach. Those who were allocated to the nonswimmers group (control group) were requested to wait on the sand for the allocated 10 minutes. Both groups were interviewed about their health, eating habits, water-contact activities, and other possible non-water-related risk factors for gastroenteritis on the day of bathing and 1 week later. The study staff were blinded to the bathing status of each person during the follow-up interview. Samples of sea water were also taken for assessment of possible contamination. By the end of data analysis, the main finding was that gastroenteritis was related to the levels of fecal streptococci if bathers had been in water at chest level.

Retrieval Can Be Done Using Any of the Following:

MeSH indexing	Clinical trial (publication type)
	Randomized controlled trial (publication type)
	Risk factors
Textwords	Randomised (title and abstract)
	Trial (abstract)

Example 4–2

Cohort study

Bosma H, Marmot MG, Hemingway H, et al. Low job control and risk of coronary heart disease in Whitehall II (prospective cohort) study. BMJ 1997;314:558–65.

This study looked at the issue of perceived job control and coronary heart disease in a large group (cohort) of civil servants. Ten thousand, three hundred and eight men and women in 20 civil service departments in London, U. K. were examined at baseline in 1985 to 1988 for the Whitehall II study. They were assessed for many factors, including psychological factors at work, especially perceived job control. The perceived job stress was evaluated so that people were put into categories of high and low job control. At 5.3

MEDLINE Record for Example 4–1

Unique Identifier   95020007

Authors   Kay D. Fleisher JM. Salmon RL. Jones F. Wyer MD. Godfree AF. Zelenauch-Jacquotte Z. Shore R.

Institution   Leeds Environment Centre, University of Leeds, UK.

Title   Predicting likelihood of gastroenteritis from sea bathing: results from **randomised** exposure.

Source   Lancet. 344(8927):905–9, 1994 Oct 1.

MeSH Subject Headings
Adult   Male
*Enterococcus/ip [Isolation & Purification]   Oceans and Seas
*Environmental Exposure/ae [Adverse Effects]   **Risk Factors**
Female   ·   Support, Non-U.S. Gov't
*Gastroenteritis/et [Etiology]   *Swimming
Human   Water Microbiology/st [Standards]
Logistic Models   *Water Microbiology

Abstract
The health effects of bathing in coastal waters is an area of scientific controversy. We conducted the first ever **randomised** "trial" of an environmental exposure to measure the health effects of this activity. The trial was spread over four summers in four UK resorts and 1216 adults took part. Detailed interviews were used to collect data on potential confounding factors and intensive water quality monitoring was used to provide more precise indices of exposure. 548 people were randomised to bathing, and the exposure included total immersion of the head. Crude rates of gastroenteritis were significantly higher in the exposed group (14.8 per 100) than the unexposed group (9.7 per 100; p = 0.01). Linear trend and multiple logistic regression techniques were used to establish relations between gastroenteritis and microbiological water quality. Of a range of microbiological indicators assayed only faecal streptococci concentration, measured at chest depth, showed a significant dose-response relation with gastroenteritis. Adverse health effects were identified when faecal streptococci concentrations exceeded 32 per 100 mL. This relation was independent of non-water-related predictors of gastroenteritis. We do not suggest that faecal streptococci caused the excess of gastrointestinal symptoms in sea bathers but these microorganisms do seem to be a better indicator of water quality than the traditional coliform counts. Bathing water standards should be revised with these findings in mind.

Publication Type   Clinical Trial. Journal Article. **Randomized Controlled Trial.**

years, the end of the follow-up of the total cohort, all participants were assessed for coronary heart disease. Final analysis, using OR, instead of the relative risks that could have been used, showed that men and women who perceived that they had low job control compared with perceived high control had an increased risk for coronary heart disease. The OR was 1.93 (95% CI 1.34 to 2.77).

Retrieval Can Use Any of the Following:

MeSH indexing	Cohort studies
	Odds ratio
	Prospective studies
	Risk factors
Textwords	Association (abstract)
	Risk (abstract)
	Prospective cohort study (abstract)
	Odds ratio

Example 4–3
Case-control study
Hippisley-Cox J, Fielding K, Pringle M. Depression as a risk factor for ischaemic heart disease in men: population based case-control study. BMJ 1998;316:1714–9.

This case-control study was designed to study the association between depression, anxiety, and use of antidepressants and ischemic heart disease in Britain. The study was done in the U. K. in one group family practice. Case patients were 188 men and 139 women with depression. Four hundred and eight-five men and 412 women who were not depressed were the control participants. (Note that not all matching is or can be done perfectly on a one-on-one basis. Sometimes half of a pair is missing, and sometimes the pairing matches one case patient with several control patients.) At the end of the study, researchers evaluated the presence of ischemic heart disease in all men and women in both groups. Men who had ischemic heart disease were almost three times more likely to have been depressed than men who did not have ischemic heart disease (OR adjusted for all confounders 2.75; 95% CI 1.13 to 6.69; $P = .03$). Depression was not a risk factor for ischemic heart disease in women using the same multivariate analysis (adjusted OR 1.34; 95% CI 0.70 to 2.56; $P=.38$). Anxiety and subsequent coronary heart disease were not significantly associated in men or women. For this case-control study, depression may be an independent risk factor for coronary heart disease in men, but not in women.

Retrieval Can Use Any of the Following:

MeSH Indexing	Case-control studies
	Risk factors
	Time factors

MEDLINE Record for Example 4–2

Unique Identifier   97208772

Authors   Bosma H. Marmot MG. Hemingway H. Nicholson AC. Brunner E. Stansfeld SA.

Institution   Department of Epidemiology and Public Health, University College London Medical School.

Title   Low job control and risk of coronary heart disease in Whitehall II (prospective cohort) study.

Source   BMJ. 314(7080):558–65, 1997 Feb 22.

MeSH Subject Headings
Adult	*Occupational Diseases/ep [Epidemiology]
Cohort Studies	Occupational Diseases/px [Psychology]
*Coronary Disease/ep [Epidemiology]	**Odds Ratio**
Coronary Disease/px [Psychology]	**Prospective Studies**
Female	Psychology, Social
Human	**Risk Factors**
London/ep [Epidemiology]	Support, Non-U.S. Gov't
Male	Support, U.S. Gov't, P.H.S.
Middle Age	

Abstract
OBJECTIVE: To determine the **association** between adverse psychosocial characteristics at work and **risk** of coronary heart disease among male and female civil servants. DESIGN: **Prospective cohort study** (Whitehall II study). At the baseline examination (1985–8) and twice during follow up a self report questionnaire provided information on psychosocial factors of the work environment and coronary heart disease. Independent assessments of the work environment were obtained from personnel managers at baseline. Mean length of follow up was 5.3 years. SETTING: London based office staff in 20 civil service departments. SUBJECTS: 10,308 civil servants aged 35-55 were examined-6895 men (67%) and 3413 women (33%). MAIN OUTCOME MEASURES: New cases of angina (Rose questionnaire), severe pain across the chest, diagnosed ischaemic heart disease, and any coronary event. RESULTS: Men and women with low job control, either self reported or independently assessed, had a higher risk of newly reported coronary heart disease during follow up. Job control assessed on two occasions three years apart, although intercorrelated, had cumulative effects on newly reported disease. Subjects with low job control on both occasions had an **odds ratio** for any subsequent coronary event of 1.93 (95% confidence interval 1.34 to 2.77) compared with subjects with high job control at both occasions. This association could not be explained by employment grade, negative affectivity, or classic coronary risk factors. Job demands and social support at work were not related to the risk of coronary heart disease. CONCLUSIONS: Low control in the work environment is associated with an increased risk of future coronary heart disease among men and women employed in government offices. The cumulative effect of low job control assessed on two occasions indicates that giving employees more variety in tasks and a stronger say in decisions about work may decrease the risk of coronary heart disease.

Publication Type   Journal Article.

This article was first published by the BMJ 1997 Feb 22; 314:558–65 and is produced by permission of the BMJ.

Textwords	Relation (abstract)
	Association (abstract)
	Adjusted odds ratio (abstract)
	Case-control study (title, abstract)
	Risk factor (title, abstract)

Example 4–4
Cross-sectional study with statistically adjusted groups

Seidman DS, Laor A, Gale R, et al. Long-term effects of vacuum and forceps deliveries. Lancet. 1991;337:1583–5.

This study was done in Israel to determine whether obstetric interventions (forceps, vacuum forceps, or cesarean section) were associated with intellectual or physical deficits in children 15 to 20 years later. The study was done in a country with socialized medicine and compulsory military draft for all 17-year-old boys and girls. Therefore, data were available from birth records (1964 to 1972) and from intelligence tests done at military entry. The raw data—data analyzed before inclusion of all possible confounding factors such as birth order, mother's age at birth of child, socioeconomic class at birth, and at military enrollment—showed that an intelligent child had most likely been delivered by forceps. In other words, if the raw data were to be believed, to obtain an intelligent child one would ask for a forceps delivery. When other factors were accounted for in the analysis, this association disappeared. The findings of the study concluded that no association existed between vacuum or forceps delivery and either physical or cognitive impairment at 17 years of age. This study shows some of the possible difficulties in designing, analyzing, and interpreting the results of etiology studies using cross-sectional studies with statistically adjusted groups instead of randomized, controlled trials or cohort or case-control studies. Researchers who work with cross-sectional studies only have one opportunity to gather their data. They do not have access to previous medical records, dietary questionnaires, or frozen blood samples, and so on, for analysis. They also do not have the time to wait until outcomes develop.

Retrieval Can Use Any of the Following:

MeSH Indexing	Comparative study
	Longitudinal studies
Textwords	Risk (abstract)
	Confounding factors (abstract)

MEDLINE Record for Example 4–3

Unique Identifier   98278738

Authors   Hippisley-Cox J. Fielding K. Pringle M.

Institution   Department of General Practice, The Medical School, Queen's Medical Centre, Nottingham NG7 2UH. julia.h-cox:nottingham.ac.uk

Title   Depression as a **risk factor** for ischaemic heart disease in men: population based case-control study.

Source   BMJ. 316(7146):1714–9, 1998 Jun 6.

MeSH Subject Headings

Adult	Female
Aged	Human
Antidepressive Agents, Tricyclic/tu	Male
[Therapeutic Use]	Middle Age
Anxiety/co [Complications]	*Myocardial Ischemia/px
	[Psychology]
Case-Control Studies	Risk Factors
*Depressive Disorder/co [Complications]	Time Factors
Depressive Disorder/dt [Drug Therapy]	

Abstract
OBJECTIVE: To determine the **relation** between depression, anxiety, and use of antidepressants and the onset of ischaemic heart disease. DESIGN: Population based **case-control study**. SETTING: All 5623 patients registered with one general practice. SUBJECTS: 188 male cases with ischaemic heart disease matched by age to 485 male controls without ischaemic heart disease; 139 female cases with ischaemic heart disease matched by age to 412 female controls. MAIN OUTCOME MEASURE: Adjusted odds ratios calculated by conditional logistic regression. RESULTS: The risk of ischaemic heart disease was three times higher among men with a recorded diagnosis of depression than among controls of the same age (**odds ratio** 3.09; 95% confidence interval 1.33 to 7.21; P=0.009). This **association** persisted when smoking status, diabetes, hypertension, and underprivileged area (UPA(8)) score were included in a multivariate model (adjusted 2.75; 1.13 to 6.69; P=0.03). Men with depression within the preceding 10 years were three times more likely to develop ischaemic heart disease than were the controls (3.13; 1.27 to 7.70; P=0.01). Men with ischaemic heart disease had a higher risk of subsequent ischaemic heart disease than men without ischaemic heart disease (adjusted 2.34; 1.34 to 4.10; P=0.003). Depression was not a **risk factor** for ischaemic heart disease in women on multivariate analysis (adjusted 1.34; 0.70 to 2.56; P=0.38). Anxiety and subsequent ischaemic heart disease were not significantly associated in men or women. CONCLUSION: Depression may be an independent risk factor for ischaemic heart disease in men, but not in women.

Publication Type   Journal Article.

This article was first published by the BMJ 1998 Jun 6;316:1714–9 and is produced by permission of the BMJ.

MEDLINE Record for Example 4–4

Unique Identifier   91269939

Authors   Seidman DS. Laor A. Gale R. Stevenson DK. Mashiach S. Danon YL.

Institution   Department of Obstetrics and Gynaecology, Sheba Medical Centre, Tel-Hashomer, Israel.

Title   Long-term effects of vacuum and forceps deliveries.

Source   Lancet. 337(8757):1583–5, 1991 Jun 29.

MeSH Subject Headings

Adolescence	Israel
Cesarean Section/ae [Adverse Effects]	Longitudinal Studies
Comparative Study	Male
*Extraction, Obstetrical	Obstetrical Forceps
Female	Pregnancy
Fetal Macrosomia/et [Etiology]	Support, Non-U.S. Gov't
Human	Vacuum Extraction, Obstetrical/ae
Infant, Low Birth Weight	[Adverse Effects]
Infant, Newborn	Wechsler Scales
*Intelligence	

Abstract
The long-term effects of vacuum and forceps deliveries are largely unknown. We determined the long-term outcome of instrumental deliveries in 52,282 infants born in Jerusalem between 1964 and 1972. For each individual, events at birth were related to results of an intelligence test and medical examination done at 17 years of age by the Israeli Defence Forces draft board. 1747 individuals were delivered by vacuum, 937 by forceps, 47,500 by spontaneous delivery, and 2098 by caesarean section. Crude data showed that mean intelligence scores at 17 were significantly higher (p less than 0.0001) in the vacuum and forceps deliveries groups than in the spontaneous-delivery group; however, after adjustment for **confounding factors** by stepwise multiple regression, these differences were no longer seen. Although the forceps-delivery group had functional impairment of feet, vision, and retina compared with the spontaneous-delivery group, and the vacuum-extraction group had impairment of the legs, differences were small. Our findings suggest that infants delivered by vacuum or forceps are not at **risk** of physical and cognitive impairment at 17 years of age.

Publication Type   Journal Article.

ASSIGNMENT

Try these searches using whatever database you think is best.

1. What does the evidence say about the possible association between secondhand smoke and cot death (SIDS or sudden infant death syndrome)?
2. Is there a proven protective effect of onions and garlic against any type of cancer or cardiovascular disease?
3. Is a family history of diabetes mellitus as strong a predictor for development of the disease as exposure to cow's milk in the first few years of life?
4. Benzodiazepines have been used for years for elderly persons for conditions such as delirium, agitation, and sleep disorders. They seem to be effective, but some have associated dangers. What does the evidence say about motor vehicle accidents?
5. Alzheimer's disease is becoming more common—maybe because the baby boomers are getting older. Find all the risk factors you can: both factors that are protective and those associated with an increased risk. Grade the evidence you find according to the following categories:

   Grade A Randomized controlled trials
   Grade B Cohort studies
   Grade C Case-control studies
   Grade D Case series (five to 20 patients and no control group)
   Grade E Case reports (one or two persons) and opinion

REFERENCES

1. Horst PA, Krombout D, Brand R. For debate: pet birds as an independent risk factor for lung cancer. BMJ 1988;297:1319–21.
2. Jadad AR. Randomised controlled trials. A user's guide. London: BMJ Books; 1998.
3. Doll R, Hill AB. Smoking and carcinoma of the lung: preliminary report. Br Med J 1950;2: 740–8.
4. Shands KN, Schmid GP, Dan BB, et al. Toxic-shock syndrome in menstruating women: association with tampon use and *Staphylococcus aureus* and clinical features in 52 cases. N Engl J Med 1980;303:1436–42.
5. Hurwitz ES, Barrett MJ, Bregman D, et al. Public Health Service study of Reye's syndrome and medications. Report of the main study. JAMA 1987;257:1905–11.
6. Salonen JT, Nyyssonen K, Korpela H, et al. High stored iron levels are associated with excess risk of myocardial infarction in eastern Finnish men. Circulation 1992;86:803–11.
7. Willett WC, Manson JE, Stampfer MJ, et al. Weight, weight change, and coronary heart disease in women. Risk within the "normal" weight range. JAMA 1995;273:461–5.
8. DiFranza JR, Lew RA. Morbidity and mortality in children associated with the use of tobacco products by other people. Pediatrics 1996;97:560–8.
9. Levine M, Walter S, Lee H, et al. for the Evidence-Based Medicine Working Group. Users' guides to the medical literature. IV. How to use an article about harm. JAMA 1994;271:1615–9.

5

Natural History and Prognosis

The last type of primary clinical research we will look at has two designations: natural history and prognosis. Traditionally, **natural history** has been considered the progression of untreated disease, and **prognosis** is the progression of treated disease. A more recent definition has natural history starting earlier in the disease process—at the time that changes start to happen at the cellular level in humans; and prognosis starts after the disease has been diagnosed. Health care professionals need to have ready access to natural history and prognosis information to respond to their patients' requests. One of the first questions patients ask when they are given a new diagnosis is, what will happen to me now? They want know the implications of their newly diagnosed disease or condition for survival, disease progression, and lifestyle, even before they start to assess treatment or palliative care options and issues.

Some epidemiologists consider that the major issue for natural history and prognosis studies is *whether* to treat: in contrast with therapy, where the issue is *how* to treat; with diagnosis, where the issue is *what* to treat; and with etiology, where the issue is *how did I get here*? A high quality prognosis and natural history study is done using a cohort study design. A group of people with a specific disease are followed over time to discover the disease progression. The patients are often newly diagnosed or at an early stage, and high follow-up is important to the quality of the study and its results.

CLINICAL EXAMPLE: GRIEF AFTER MISCARRIAGE

A good example of a natural history and prognosis study was done in the Netherlands. Janssen et al.[1] were interested in documenting women's experiences during pregnancy and after birth. They asked readers of a popular family magazine who were in the early stages of pregnancy to volunteer for their study, which included a series of questionnaires about the pregnancy and delivery, and about the child's first 18 months. Two thousand, one hundred and forty women volunteered, and 227 subsequently had a miscarriage. This group of women was studied separately for up to 18 months after the miscarriage to learn about the natural grieving process and what factors predicted excessive grief, and to identify women who might need extra help getting through it. Eight-nine percent of the women who miscarried were included in the final analysis. Outcomes confirmed what common sense already tells us: grief follows miscarriage; time heals; and some women, especially those more vulnerable or without support, may need additional help. The study was well-done. The cohort was gathered before the event and followed for a reasonable time (18 months) to collect data on both short- and long-term outcomes. Questionnaire data on the issues around conception and early pregnancy were collected before the miscarriage, and therefore were not as likely to be biased by knowledge of it. Follow-up was more than 80%—another quality indicator.

Very few high quality natural history or prognosis studies are published in the literature. They are time consuming to do well, often taking many years to complete because of disease progression patterns. For example, some multiple sclerosis studies have reported data for 30 years or more, and an ongoing study of optic neuritis done by the Mayo Clinic in Minnesota[2] has 50-year data for some patients.

HOW NATURAL HISTORY AND PROGNOSIS STUDIES ARE DONE

All patients, regardless of their disease, want to know its implications. Some diseases and conditions do not need treatment, or current treatments have not proved beneficial (for example, the common cold, chicken pox, and to some extent, multiple sclerosis). Some diseases and conditions need immediate, active treatment: major hemorrhage, peptic ulcers, myocardial infarction, and appendicitis. For some, if not all, diseases it is important for the patient and health care professional to come to a decision on whether to pursue treatment. A classic and important example that demands balance between the disease progression characteristics and treatment options is the child with a slight-to-moderate degree of scoliosis. Children with scoliosis (curvature of the spine) can be crippled, or even die, if they are not treated in an appropriate and timely manner. Several effective therapies exist, but they are unpleasant and invasive, involving surgery and long-term body casts. Not all children with scoliosis, however, need treatment. Good prognosis information exists to help clinicians, patients, and families make wise decisions on a case-by-case basis.

NATURAL HISTORY VERSUS PROGNOSIS

Natural history and prognosis, although related, are not equivalent concepts. To reiterate, natural history has traditionally been considered to follow untreated disease to see what happens over time. Because multiple sclerosis has few effective treatments, natural history studies can be done; although this is changing with the introduction of new drugs, including β-interferon. Probably the best-known natural history study is the Tuskegee Study of Untreated Syphilis in the Negro Male.[3] It was started in 1931, and enrolled 399 African-American men with tertiary syphilis and 201 uninfected men, and followed them, while withholding treatment, until 1972. This study was obviously unethical and should never have never been done. Allowing untreated disease to progress when even marginally effective treatments are available is unacceptable: science must never be allowed to come before ethics, human dignity, and common sense.

Prognosis has traditionally been considered the study of treated disease over time. For example, stroke is a common disease that is treated in the hospital and at home with a variety of medical, nursing, physiotherapeutic, occupational therapy, and at times, psychological interventions. The Oxfordshire Community Stroke Project study[4] is a good example of a prognosis study. It assessed outcomes after a first-ever stroke in 675 patients who were followed for up to 6.5 years. The Oxfordshire data showed that mortality after stroke was 19% in the first 30 days and 31% in the first year. Mortality in the subsequent years decreased substantially.

The more current distinction between natural history and prognosis is that natural history starts at the biologic onset of disease and includes the periods when early diagnosis (with no symptoms) is possible, through to the time when usual clinical diagnosis occurs, to final outcome assessment. This is a four-stage process, with the first stage being very difficult, if not impossible, to realize.

Prognosis includes the time from clinical diagnosis through to outcome assessment (the two final stages of natural history). A natural history study of myocardial infarction for example, would start with the development of atherosclerosis; a prognosis study would start at the onset of chest pain.

INCEPTION COHORT STUDIES

The key issue in studying the natural history and prognosis of diseases is the collection of a *representative* sample of patients with the disease or disorder who are at an *early* stage in their disease process. Researchers assess these patients over time. This type of design is called an **inception cohort**. "Inception" means early, or at least at a uniform point in time for the disease; and "cohort" means following a group of people forward in time—just as it did for the etiology and causation studies.

When studying natural history or prognosis, it is important to identify and include patients as near to the onset of the disease as possible. This is especially true for diseases that have serious outcomes near the onset, such as stroke and bacterial meningitis. As another example, people with a myocardial infarction can die within minutes, so that studying prognosis in these patients needs to start as early as possible: probably at the front door of the emergency room, if not in the ambulance, with a check at the coroner's office for sudden deaths. Starting in the coronary care unit or a step-down unit would not truly reflect the important considerations that need to be addressed when studying the myocardial infarction disease process.

Completeness of follow-up is important for natural history and prognosis studies, as it is for therapy studies: "missing" persons can obscure the disease process. For example, a study of the progression of rheumatoid arthritis in patients who were newly diagnosed and followed in a tertiary care clinic might lose patients who had little or no disease progression: in other words, following only those patients who returned for follow-up of their rheumatoid arthritis would tend to overestimate the morbidity associated with the disease. In contrast, a study of men with advanced prostate cancer that did not include an aggressive follow-up process might "lose" men who had died. This loss would tend to show that the prognosis of prostate cancer was better than it truly is. Again, 80% is the "magic" number for follow-up that is assumed for good quality natural history and prognosis studies. Higher levels are desirable, and lower levels of follow-up rates are unacceptable.

Treatment studies using a randomized controlled trial design are another category of research that can also give good, reliable prognosis information, especially for diseases with specific treatments, such as congestive heart failure. They can provide survival rates and disease progression data for the study groups or the placebo groups. Searchers need to recognize this source of information for comprehensive searching on prognosis topics.

CALCULATIONS

No special calculations or statistics are involved in natural history or prognosis studies. Quite often the reported data are similar to etiology and causation statistics and data presentation, with rates for disease progression, and specific outcomes, and the risk for these outcomes, reported. For example, Principe et al.[5] reported on 322 adults who had had a minor stroke and were followed for 10 years. Ninety-six deaths occurred, along with 69 new cerebrovascular events. Hazards ratios showed that a previous myocardial infarction increased their risk for dying by 1.8 times (hazards ratio 1.8, 95% CI 1.1 to 3.1).

SUMMARY

In summary, natural history and prognosis studies are done using an inception cohort design. Patients with a specific disease or condition are identified at diagnosis, soon after diagnosis, or at a uniform time in the disease process, and followed for an appropriate period of time in relation to that disease's process. A high follow-up (> 80% is essential) is important.

The Evidence-Based Medicine Working Group, in their *Users' Guides to the Literature*, have ranked the attributes of natural history and prognosis studies in order of importance for clinicians.[6]

- Well-defined sample of patients at a similar point in the course of the disease.
- Length and completeness of follow-up.
- Objective and unbiased outcomes criteria
- Adjustment for important prognostic factors.

Indexing is done to reflect the cohort study design, but not for the inception aspect or for follow-up. Prognosis is indexed more often than natural history. Time factors and disease progression are also important index words. *Morbidity*, loosely defined as all the "bad things" that can happen to you except death, is not used as appropriately as possible. This is because morbidity is such a general term, and where possible indexers must index in specific terms. For example, a prognosis study of severe head injuries that assessed long-term headaches, vision disturbances, mood changes, and seizures would be indexed using terms for all five outcomes, and not a general term such as "morbidity". Author textwords are usually consistent across time and studies—"prognosis" or "prognostic," "natural history," and "cohort studies." Sometimes authors use the term *course* as in, "the clinical course of recurrent otitis media." The textword "course" has so many other meanings, such as course textbooks, course versus fine measurement, and so on that the term is not useful for retrieving only high quality prognosis studies with few irrelevant studies mixed in. Possible indexing terms and phrases for all four databases are on the following pages.

MEDLINE

MeSH, Subheadings, and Textwords for Prognosis Studies

MeSH

Cohort studies*
    Longitudinal studies
        Follow-up studies
        Prospective studies

Prognosis* (not used often enough by indexers)
    Treatment outcome
        Medical futility
        Treatment failure

Morbidity
    Incidence (number of new cases in a given period of time)
    Prevalence (number of current cases in a certain area)

Mortality*
    Cause of death
    Infant mortality
    Maternal mortality
    Survival rate

Survival analysis
Disease susceptibility
Disease progression*
Disease-free survival
Time factors*
Recurrence

Subheadings
Mortality
Diagnosis (more useful in back files)

Textwords
natural history*
inception cohort
predict:
prognostic factor
prognos:*
clinical course
outcome
course

---

*indicates a preferred term

CINAHL Database of Nursing and Allied Health Literature

CINAHL Index Terms, Subheadings, and Document Types for Prognosis Studies

CINAHL Index Terms
Prospective studies
    Concurrent prospective studies
    Nonconcurrent prospective studies
    Pseudolongitudinal studies
    Panel studies
        Retrospective panel studies
        Revolving panel studies
Prognosis
    Outcomes (health care)
        Medical futility
        Nursing outcomes
        Outcome assessment
        Outcomes of prematurity
        Pregnancy outcomes
        Treatment outcomes
            Treatment failure
Morbidity
    Incidence
    Prevalence
Mortality
    Child mortality
    Hospital mortality
    Infant mortality
    Maternal mortality
    Perinatal mortality

Survival analysis
    Cox proportional hazards model
    Kaplan-Meier estimator
    Log-rank test
Disease progression
Recurrence
Non-experimental research
    Case-control studies
        Hospital-based case control
        Matched case control
        Population based case control
    Correlational studies
    Prospective studies
        Concurrent prospective studies
        Nonconcurrent prospectiave studies
        Panel studies
            Retrospective panel studies
            Revolving panel studies
        Pseudolongitudinal studies

Subheadings
Mortality
Diagnosis
Prognosis
Symptoms

Document types
Research

Textwords
Use same list as for MEDLINE

CINAHL thesaurus terms selected by Katy Nesbit
All extracts from the CINAHL® Thesaurus Copyright © 1999, Cinahl Information Systems. Reprinted with permission from Cinahl Information Systems.

PsycINFO

Descriptors, Publication Types, and Textwords for Prognosis

Descriptors
Death and Dying
Prognosis

Disease Course
Treatment Effectiveness Evaluation
Treatment Outcomes
Psychotherapeutic Outcomes
Recovery (Disorders)
Relapse (Disorders)

Remission (Disorders)+
    Spontaneous Remission
    Symptom Remission

Quality of Life
Psychosocial Factors
Sociocultural Factors+

Methodology Descriptors
Cohort Analysis
Content Analysis
Data Collection

Empirical Methods+
Experimental Methods
    Observation Methods

Meta Analysis
Self Report
Between Groups Design
Follow-up Studies
Longitudinal Studies
Repeated Measures
Experiment Controls (Used for Control groups)

Textwords
Cohort Stud:*
Prospective Stud:*
Morbidity
Incidence
Prevalence
Mortality
Cause of Death
Survival rate
Disease progression
Time factor:*
Natural history
Inception Cohort:*

Prognostic factor:*
Clinical course
Outcome
Course
Disease Free Survival
Cure

Publication Type or Form/Content Type
Empirical Study
Followup Study
Longitudinal Study
Meta Analysis
Prospective Study
Treatment Outcome Study

+ indicates term can be exploded
*indicates preferred term
PsycINFO terms selected by Jean Sullivant

EMBASE/EXCERPTA MEDICA

Index Terms, Links, and EMTAGS for Natural History and Prognosis Studies

Index terms
Cohort analysis
Incidence
    Cancer incidence
    Familial incidence
    Parasitic incidence
Morbidity
    Maternal morbidity
        Chiari frommel syndrome
        Maternal disease
        Postpartum hemorrhage
        Puerperal depression
        Puerperal infection
        Puerperal psychosis
    Perinatal mortality
        Newborn mortality
    Mortality
        Cancer mortality
        Prenatal mortality
        Surgical mortality

   Childhood mortality
   Embryo mortality
   Fetus morality
   Infant mortality
   Maternal mortality
   Perinatal mortality
      Newborn mortality
Prevalance [do not explode]
Survival
   Cancer survival
   Life expectancy
   Survival rate
   Survival time
Disease course
   Acute disease
   Cancer growth
   Cancer inhibition
   Cancer recurrence
   Cancer regression
   Chronic disease
   Chronicity
   Convalescence
   Deterioration
   Disease duration
   Incubation time
   Leukemia remission
   Metastasis inhibition
   Onset age
   Prognosis
   Recurrent disease
   Reinfection
   Relapse
   Remission
   Reversal reaction
   Terminal disease
   Tumor growth
   Tumor recurrence
   Tumor regression
   Survival
      Cancer survival
      Life expectancy
      Survival rate
      Survival time

Disease severity
    Acute disease
    Advanced cancer
    Cancer size
    Chronic disease
    Critical illness
    Deterioration
    Prognosis
    Terminal disease

Links (subheadings)
    Epidemiology

Emtags (publication types)
    Sex differences
    Ethnic or racial aspects
    Epidemiology

MEDLINE HEDGES

MEDLINE hedges have been constructed for natural history and prognosis studies. The best single term is:

exp cohort studies (MeSH)

The best complex search strategy with the highest sensitivity is:

**incidence (MeSH)
OR explode mortality (MeSH)
OR follow-up studies (MeSH)
OR mortality (subheading)
OR prognos: (textword)
OR predict: (textword)
OR course (textword)**

The complex search strategy with the highest specificity is:

**prognosis (MeSH)
OR survival analysis (MeSH)**

Example 5–1
Natural History Example
Barnhart HX, Caldwell MB, Thomas P, et al. Natural history of human immunodeficiency virus disease in perinatally infected children: an analysis from the Pediatric Spectrum of Disease Project. Pediatrics 1996;97:710–6.

This study from Emory University in Atlanta is an example of a well-done natural history study. It studied infants of women who were HIV-positive. Researchers wanted to know how HIV-disease progressed in infants who became HIV-positive. Starting in 1982, 2148 children were studied. They were assessed every 6 months from birth until 1993. They lived in seven geographic regions of the U. S. and Puerto Rico. By the end of 1993, 458 (21%) children had died, 17% had severe symptoms, 54% had moderate symptoms, 7% had mild symptoms, and 2% had no symptoms. Overall, children progressed to moderate symptoms in their second year of life, and their mean age at death was 9.4 years. This study is one of the few true natural history studies available. Children were included in the study before they became HIV-positive and were followed until death. Follow-up was good. The results may no longer be valid, however, as more and better medications that can prevent and treat HIV infection have been developed since 1982.

Retrieval Can Use Any of the Following:

MeSH indexing	Cause of death
	Comparative study
	Disease progression
	Survival rate
	Time factors
textwords	Natural history (abstract and title)
	Progression (abstract)

Example 5–2
Prognosis Example
Brancati FL, Chow JW, Wagener MM, et al. Is pneumonia really the old man's friend? Two-year prognosis after community-acquired pneumonia. Lancet 1993;342:30–3.

This study was done in a Veterans' Affairs hospital in Pennsylvania. It looks at the predictors of in-hospital and 2-year death in patients hospitalized with community-acquired pneumonia. It also assesses whether pneumonia should be treated in the elderly. In some cultures, pneumonia is called the "old man's friend" and it is untreated because death from pneumonia can be easier than death from other diseases. In contrast, some cultures treat pneumonia in patients in all situations, even when some consideration could be given to nontreatment. One hundred and forty-one patients who had community-acquired pneumonia in two U.S. urban teaching hospitals were studied, starting in the hospital and ending 2 years later. Chart audit and mail and telephone surveys were used to assess mortality. Follow-up was 92% at 2 years; 22 patients (16%) died in the hospital, and another 38

MEDLINE Record for Example 5–1

Unique Identifier   96206307

Authors   Barnhart HX. Caldwell MB. Thomas P. Mascola L. Ortiz I. Hsu HW. Schulte J. Parrott R. Maldonado Y. Byers R.

Institution   Department of Biostatistics, Rollins School of Public Health, Emory University, Atlanta, Georgia 30322, USA.

Title   **Natural history** of human immunodeficiency virus disease in perinatally infected children: an analysis from the Pediatric Spectrum of Disease Project.

Source   Pediatrics. 97(5):710–6, 1996 May.

MeSH Subject Headings

Acquired Immunodeficiency Syndrome/cl [Classification]	**Disease Progression**
Acquired Immunodeficiency Syndrome/cn [Congenital]	Health Planning
	Human
Acquired Immunodeficiency Syndrome/pp [Physiopathology]	HIV Infections/cl [Classification]
Cause of Death	*HIV Infections/cn [Congenital]
Centers for Disease Control and Prevention (U.S.)	*HIV Infections/pp [Physiopathology]
	Infant
Child	Infant, Newborn
Child, Preschool	Models, Statistical
Clinical Trials	Population Surveillance
Comparative Study	Research Design
Confidence Intervals	Support, U.S. Gov't, P.H.S.
Counseling	**Survival Rate**
	Time Factors
	United States

Abstract

OBJECTIVE. To describe the **progression** of human immunodeficiency virus (HIV) disease through clinical stages from birth to death among a large number of perinatally infected children. METHODS. The Pediatric Spectrum of Disease (PSD) project, coordinated by the Centers for Disease Control and Prevention (CDC), has conducted active surveillance for HIV disease since 1988 in seven geographic regions. PSD data are collected from medical and social service records every 6 months through practitioners at each participating hospital clinic. We analyzed data from perinatally HIV-infected children born between 1982 and 1993. The **natural history** of HIV disease was divided into five progressive stages using the clinical categories in the CDC 1994 pediatric HIV classification system: stage N, no signs or symptoms; stage A, mild signs or symptoms; stage B, moderate signs or symptoms; stage C, severe signs or symptoms; and stage D, death. A five-stage Markov model was fitted to the PSD data. To compare the estimates from the PSD project with the published estimates, we also fitted an alternative Markov model using acquired immunodeficiency syndrome (AIDS; 1987 case definition) ...

Publication Type   Journal Article. Multicenter Study.

MEDLINE Record for Example 5–2

Unique Identifier   93302403

Authors   Brancati FL. Chow JW. Wagener MM. Vacarello SJ. Yu VL.

Institution   Welch Center for Prevention, Epidemiology, and Clinical Research, Johns Hopkins Medical Institutions, Baltimore, Maryland.

Title   Is pneumonia really the old man's friend? Two-year **prognosis** after community-acquired pneumonia [see comments].

Source   Lancet. 342(8862):30–3, 1993 Jul 3.

MeSH Subject Headings

Adolescence	Male
Adult	Middle Age
Age Factors	Multivariate Analysis
Aged	Pneumonia/mi [Microbiology]
Aged, 80 and over	*Pneumonia/mo [Mortality]
Cohort Studies	*Pneumonia/th [Therapy]
Comorbidity	Probability
Female	**Prognosis**
Follow-Up Studies	**Prospective Studies**
Hematocrit	**Risk**
Hospital Mortality	Socioeconomic Factors
Hospitalization	Support, U.S. Gov't, P.H.S.
Human	**Survival Rate**

Abstract

Is pneumonia "the old man's friend"—a terminal event for patients who will otherwise die soon of underlying chronic disease? If so, chronological age might influence treatment policy. We investigated the predictors of 2-year mortality after patients' admission to hospital for community-acquired pneumonia, and focused on the predictive value of age. In a **prospective cohort study** 141 consecutive patients were admitted to hospital with community-acquired pneumonia. Clinical, laboratory, and sociodemographic data were collected on admission. Comorbidity was categorised as mild, moderate, or severe by a physician based on the patient's medical history. **Survival** was assessed at 24 months after discharge. 22 (16%) patients died in hospital. Of the remaining 119, 38 (32%) died over the next 24 months. In a Cox model, 2-year **mortality** was independently related to severe comorbidity (**relative risk** [RR] = 9.4) or moderate comorbidity (RR = 3.1), and to haematocrit less than 35% (RR = 2.9) (all $p <$ or = to 0.005). However, compared with patients aged 18–44 years, patients aged 45–64 (RR = 0.84), 65–74 (RR = 1.28), and 75–92 (RR = 1.99) were not significantly more likely to die during the 24 months after discharge (all $p >$ or = to 0.2). Old age should not be a sole criterion for withholding aggressive treatment of community-acquired pneumonia.

Publication Type   Journal Article.

(32%) died in the next two years. The biggest predictor of mortality was comorbidity, and the prognosis for older patients was not necessarily worse than for younger patients. No evidence was found that pneumonia should routinely go untreated in elderly patients.

Retrieval Can Use Any of the Following:

MeSH Indexing	Age factors
	Cohort studies
	Follow-up studies
	Prognosis
	Prospective studies
	Risk
	Survival rate
Textwords	Prognosis (title)
	Prospective cohort study (abstract)
	Survival (abstract)
	Relative risk (abstract)
	Mortality (abstract)

ASSIGNMENT

1. Is optic neuritis a risk factor for the development of multiple sclerosis? What is the risk by decade (for example, 10, 20, 30, 40-year risk)?

2. Persons who have ulcerative colitis have been told for decades that they have an increased risk for developing colorectal cancer. Is this statement true? Is ulcerative colitis a bigger risk for colorectal cancer than a family history of colorectal cancer?

3. Delirium in hospitalized patients used to be thought of as a benign condition. Use the literature to deterimine whether this is true, especially for elderly patients.

4. What are the risk factors for recurrence of a first seizure in adults? What are the risk factors for recurrence of a first seizure in infants? (*Hint:* these are two separate searches.) Are any of the risk factors the same?

5. Adolescents have many things to cope with as they go through high school and get ready for university. Learning how to live with chronic disease can be difficult for anyone, and especially so for adolescents. Is the rate of depression higher in teens who develop either type 1 or type 2 diabetes mellitus than for teens who do not develop diabetes mellitus?

REFERENCES

1. Janssen HJ, Cuisinier MC, de Graauw KP, et al. A prospective study of risk factors predicting grief intensity following pregnancy loss. Arch Gen Psychiatry 1997;54:56–61.
2. Rodriguez M, Siva A, Cross SA, et al. Optic neuritis: a population based study in Olmsted County, Minnesota. Neurology 1995;45:244–50.
3. Brawley OW. The study of untreated syphilis in the Negro male. Int J Radiat Oncol Biol Phys 1998;40:5–8.
4. Dennis MS, Burn JP, Sandercock PA, et al. Long-term survival after first-ever stroke: The Oxfordshire Community Stroke Project. Stroke 1993;24:796–800.
5. Principe M, Caluasso F, Rasura M, et al. Long-term prognosis after a minor stroke. 10 year mortality and major stroke recurrence in a hospital based cohort. Stroke 1998;29:126–32.
6. Laupacis A, Wells G, Richardson S, Tugwell P for the Evidence-Based Medicine Working Group. Users' guides to the medical literature. V. How to use and article about prognosis. JAMA 1994;272:234–7.

6

Secondary Publications: Systematic Review Articles

We have completed our summary of the primary EBHC studies of therapy, diagnosis, etiology and causation, and natural history and prognosis. The order in which we considered them reflects their respective prevalence in the health care literature. To complete our understanding of the types of evidence most useful to EBHC practitioners, we turn to **secondary publications**. They are called "secondary publications" because researchers take data from previously published or unpublished studies, summarize and analyze the combined results, draw conclusions, and publish their results as systematic review articles, clinical practice guidelines, and economic analyses. Many clinicians believe that a synthesis of several original studies is a better, more powerful publication with greater potential influence on clinical decisions than a single study. Many start their searches for evidence to support their EBHC quests with a strategy to retrieve a systematic review article.

SYSTEMATIC REVIEW ARTICLES AND META-ANALYSES

Evidence-based health care has embraced and further developed a new type of review article, called a **systematic review** *article*. It is similar to conventional review articles (also called a narrative review) in many respects, but differs on at least two major points. The "new" review article is based explicitly on systematic review of evidence, rather than on haphazard review of the evidence mixed inextricably with opinion. Traditional review articles often are more narrative, and have not used numerical or other cross-study analyses to synthesize the findings of original studies and come to a clinical "bottom" or conclusion. Traditional review articles are often more useful for understanding a new or complex topic. Students appreciate traditional or narrative review articles, as they are often closer to being textbook chapters that summarize a broad topic, such as the use of α- and β-interferons and how they are changing the practice of management of neurologic disease. Systematic reviews are often more clinically based, and are done to answer a narrower and more focused clinical topic, such as: what is the effectiveness (do they work in the "real" world?) and safety shown across primary studies of β-interferon to prevent relapses in multiple sclerosis?

Systematic review articles must clearly state why the review is being done: the purpose. For example, Tryba[1] completed a systematic review with the explicit purpose of evaluating the efficacy (do they work in an "ideal" world?) of antacids, H_2-antagonists, pirenzepine, and sucralfate in preventing stress ulcer bleeding, and they compared the incidence (new cases) of pneumonia and death in adults who received these agents while they were in an intensive care unit. This requirement of having an explicit statement of purpose is similar to primary studies, in that any study must define and establish the research question before the research starts.

Moreover, the methods used to find the primary studies (for example, search strategies, review of bibliographies of other review articles, and contact with the authors of important, relevant studies) must be described. To illustrate this, the following description of the retrieval process was included by Hatala et al.[2] in their systematic review article:

> "Studies were identified by searching MEDLINE (1966 to April 1995) using the keywords aminoglycosides (exploded), drug administration schedule, and adult. Additional articles were identified by hand searching of selected infectious disease journals from November 1994 to April 1995 and by scanning bibliographies of review articles, position papers, and identified articles. Primary authors of selected articles were also contacted to obtain a list of potentially relevant articles."

With provision of the search strategy information we can, if we choose, replicate the search process and examine the evidence (original studies) that the authors used to analyze, draw their conclusions, and make recommendations. Without the search strategy information we cannot distinguish fact and fiction, evidence and speculation.

History of Systematic Review Articles

The systematic review methodology was developed and refined in the disciplines of education and psychology in the late 1960s and early 1970s, although some early examples exist in the health care literature. The earliest example was published in 1904 in the *British Medical Journal* by Pearson. He presented combined data on enteric fever inoculations[3] from data provided by the British Army in India and South Africa. Another classic paper was published by Goldberger[4] in the *Bulletin of the Hygienic Laboratory* in 1907. It combined data on transmission rates of typhoid using data in reports published from 1881 to 1906. One of the more influential developers of systematic review methods in the social sciences was G. V. Glass, whose 1981 textbook is still used.[5] Glass was also the first to use the term "meta-analysis." Researchers in health care quickly found that this methodology was useful to answer clinical questions. One of the first well-done systematic reviews was by Linus Pauling on the usefulness of vitamin C in relation to the common cold.[6] He built on the research coming out of Minnesota in the late 1930s and early 1940s. This systematic review indicated that vitamin C could help ward off the common cold and reduce symptoms if a cold developed, but the data are still inconclusive, and research continues sporadically throughout the world. Tom Chalmers, considered to be one of the founders and developers of the systematic review methodology in health care, used Pauling's systematic review as the basis of his 1975 trial on vitamin C that was funded by the U.S. National Institutes of Health—the same one referred to in our introduction, that involved patients who ascertained if they were taking vitamin C or sugar.

Other Names

Systematic reviews have historically been given many names, which is consistent with any new and developing area, especially one that develops across disciplines and continents. These various names are important for retrieval of systematic review articles, especially the reviews that were published before indexers started to recognize them as systematic reviews and provide appropriate index terms. For MEDLINE, the publication types that make retrieval of certain types of articles, including meta-analyses, much easier were introduced in 1991. Systematic review articles have been called:

> systematic review or overview
> meta-analysis
> metaanalysis
> meta analysis
> metanalysis
> met-analysis
> meta-analytic review or overview
> quantitative review or overview
> quantitative synthesis
> integrative review or overview
> integrative research review or overview
> research integration or overview
> collaborative review or overview
> methodologic or methodological review or overview
> meta-regression
> metaregression
> mega-regression

Overview Versus Review

Geography tends to dictate the use of the two terms *review* and *overview*. An overview done in Europe and the British Commonwealth countries tends to be called "a systematic review article" whereas in the U.S. an "overview" is often a narrative (traditional) review article. For example, the study by Macharia et al.[7] was done in Canada, and it is definitely a systematic review that collects and synthesizes the evidence on improving patient appointment keeping. The bottom line is that appointment keeping can be increased, but it takes time and effort, and may include telephone calls, mailed individualized reminders, and contracting with the patients. In contrast, the paper by Wattenberg[8] published in the U.S. is very much a narrative review of chemoprevention, with no description of how the literature used was chosen. No current searching technique can be used to tell which category of "overview" a given study belongs to: only a reading of the methods section of each one can identify which overview is a systematic review article and which one is a narrative review article.

Why Are Systematic Reviews Done?

A systematic review is done for five major reasons:

1. To get to a "bottom line" using all studies on a topic. More than one study may have been done on a question or a closely related question. For example, there is no definite conclusion about the maximum amount of time after onset of symptoms that thrombolytic therapy should be administered to patients with myocardial infarction. Systematic reviews have been done and analysis across studies shows that as soon as possible after symptoms start is the ideal time to start thrombolysis, and a natural maximum time seems to exist beyond which the treatment no longer provides benefit. The evidence seems to suggest this may be in the range of 6 hours after symptom onset.

2. To increase the precision of estimates of the effects of a treatment, of etiology and causation, or of another topic. Precise estimates of the effect of an intervention often need to be calculated statistically using several hundred incidents or outcomes. The study by Frick et al.[9] that we used in the therapy chapter assessed the rate of myocardial infarction in men with high levels of cholesterol. Approximately 2.5% of the men in the study had a heart attack during the 5-year follow-up. If we needed 250 "events," or myocardial infarctions, before we could come to a precise estimate of the effect of the drug gemfibrozil, we would need to study 10,000 men. Although a study of this size is possible, it is improbable that it would be financed by routine funding agencies. As an alternative to the large study, we can use the studies on gemfibrozil already published, complete a meta-analysis of the data, and come to a more precise estimate without enrolling a single new patient.

3. To increase the number of patients in clinically relevant subgroups. For example, studies of patients with heart problems may include a small proportion with diabetes mellitus. By combining data across several studies for patients with diabetes, researchers can more fully evaluate the effect of the comorbidities (diabetes and acute coronary syndromes). Also, the condition or disease may be sufficiently rare that it is difficult to assemble enough patients to study, even when using more than one clinical center or city for recruitment.

4. To resolve discrepancies in findings. Small studies of similar interventions in similar patients can have conflicting results. Either a larger study or systematic review of the already-published studies may provide the definitive answer.

5. To plan new studies. Granting agencies often require a formal calculation of the needed numbers of patients to test a study hypothesis. A meta-analysis is becoming the standard method of doing this calculation and of providing data for the funding proposal or granting agency.

Steps

Producing a systematic review is a time- and resource-intensive process. Although the systematic review process is still being developed, the production involves five specific steps. Any review article produced using these steps is considered to be a systematic review article:

1. Problem formulation.
2. Identification and selection articles for inclusion.
3. Data extraction for analysis.
4. Analysis and statistical confirmation.
5. Presentation of results.

Step 1: Problem Formulation

Problem formulation must include not only the question but also the interventions, populations, settings, outcomes, duration, and the inclusion and exclusion criteria for the individual studies. The purpose sets the stage for the next steps, especially the literature step process.

Step 2: Identifying and Selecting Studies for Inclusion

As the systematic review methodology matures, the second step is becoming more rigorous. Some early online searches involved two or three term searches (for example, screening and colorectal neoplasia: neither of which is an index term in MEDLINE). The first part of this step often includes some of the following techniques or processes:

- Searching multiple general and specific bibliographic and other funding, research, educational, and other databases.
- Complex, multifaceted searching strategies using index terms, textwords, and other database-specific techniques.
- Citation searching using *Science Citation Index* or *Social Sciences Citation Index* to determine which new articles have included the relevant studies and review articles in their bibliographies (that is, which new studies have cited this important study that I have identified?).
- Hand searches of specific journals.
- Hand searches of conference proceedings and meeting abstracts
- Contact with authors and other experts in the field.
- Contact with professional organizations and government departments, including the U.S. Centers for Disease Control and Prevention, and other, similar, national reporting agencies.
- Contact with manufacturers.
- Scanning bibliographies of review articles, selected studies, book chapters, clinical practice guidelines, and theses.
- Using PubMed (a MEDLINE searching system from the National Library of Medicine) to retrieve articles that it determines are related in content.

Often, the searching process starts with a comprehensive search for narrative and systematic review articles before searching for primary studies. This not only verifies that a systematic review has not been done on the topic, but their bibliographies also provide citations for the new systematic review.

Much discussion has concerned how best to collect all the relevant studies for combination into a systematic review. Published studies are the easiest to collect. Studies in other categories, often called the *gray literature* are much more difficult to collect. The gray literature includes unpublished internal company research reports, preliminary works, studies done only for submission to national drug approval agencies, preliminary studies done before a full study to check the process and procedures, and studies that have not yet been published or submitted for publication. This last category is important for persons who want to produce comprehensive systematic review articles. Researchers, journal peer reviewers, and editors, being human, prefer to publish studies that have positive results (that is, that show a difference: the drug or other intervention is shown to be effective). Studies with negative results (that is, that do not show a difference: the proposed surgery is no better than the standard procedure we already use) have been shown to be submitted less often for publication, be submitted longer after completion of the study, be rejected more often by journal editors, and be published in less well known or in less respected journals than studies with "positive" results. If identification of these negative trials is not pursued, systematic review of studies can tend to overemphasize the true direction and magnitude of the combined results.

Drug companies fund many studies of their new products. Researchers employed or funded by the companies may be encouraged not to publish negative trials. This fact may also lead to meta-analyses that do not include all possible trials, and that can, therefore, be over-optimistic.

After potential studies are identified by computer and hand searching, each one is examined to ascertain whether it fits the inclusion criteria and does not meet any of the exclusion criteria set by the author. The following set of inclusion and exclusion criteria comes from a meta-analysis by Schneider and Olin[10] (they called it an "overview") on the use of hydergine for treating dementia. Their inclusion and exclusion criteria for selecting articles for analysis are listed below. Frequently, more than one person reviews the potential studies for inclusion and exclusion to ensure that the process is rigorous and reproducible.

Inclusion Criteria
- Hydergine was used to treat elderly patients.
- Patients had possible cognitive impairment or dementia.
- Each study was a randomized controlled trial.

Exclusion Criteria
- Treatment duration was not described.
- The trial was not double-blind or placebo-controlled.
- The trial was either a crossover trial without first-period data, or an open trial.
- Hydergine was administered intravenously.
- The patient sample was inappropriate.

- Outcomes were inadequately reported.
- End-points were nonclinical (for example, blood levels of the drug).
- The outcome was reported elsewhere.

Step 3: Extraction of Data

The third step is the extraction of the data from the studies. The data from each study are put into a tabular format to: help the reviewer understand the range of studies included; assess the data for possible combination (meta-analysis); and provide the raw data for the statistical calculations in the next step, and formal presentation for publication. This step is important, and often difficult to complete accurately and consistently. Therefore, researchers often complete this task in duplicate or even triplicate, compare their results for consistency, and reconcile their differences themselves or bring in a third or fourth party to arbitrate. In many systematic reviews data are extracted from studies that have met the selection criteria for most or all of the following:

- Patient numbers and characteristics at baseline.
- Study quality (poor quality studies often seem to have "better" results than similar, higher quality studies).
- Study intervention characteristics, including drug, dose, duration, administration route, and so on.
- Follow-up duration and numbers.
- Outcomes and how these are defined and assessed.
- Confounders or other risk factors.
- Adverse effects.
- The country where the study was done and published.
- The year of publication.

Step 4: Analysis and Statistical Confirmation

At step 4 researchers determine, using both clinical common sense and statistical computations, whether the data are *similar* enough—with respect to: study participants; interventions, including doses and medications; outcome measures; and character of results—for the data to be combined mathematically and statistically. If the studies and data are similar enough the studies are considered to have *homogeneity*, and the data are pooled and analyzed together, using special meta-analytic techniques and programs. If the individual studies show *heterogeneity*, they are not similar enough for combining, and no further statistical analysis should be done using the data from the studies.

At this point, if the data can be combined, the systematic review article becomes a meta-analysis. **Meta-analysis** is a subcategory of systematic review articles, and therefore, although it is called a "meta-analysis," it is also a systematic review article. Meta-analyses can be further subdivided into two categories. If the data from each *study* are combined, the resulting report is considered to be a meta-analysis. Alternatively, if the researchers, often called *meta-analysts*, go to the investigators of each of the original studies and collect and analyze data from *each patient in each trial*, the meta-analysis is often called a *collaborative review* using individual patient data.

This distinction is important both for understanding the process and for retrievals. The differences among three types of systematic reviews are illustrated using data from a systematic review by Hoffman et al.[11] published in the *Cochrane Library*. The authors collected trials of all antihypertensive medications in patients with diabetes mellitus. Patients with diabetes have a high incidence of hypertension, and it is an important risk factor for cardiovascular complications. Many trials have studied all persons with hypertension, but few have included only patients with diabetes mellitus. Instead of finding their own funding and patients, Hoffman et al. collected all the large studies of antihypertension medications they could find and extracted the data on the patients with diabetes from each study.

The following six studies evaluating the long-term use of any antihypertensive agent to reduce high blood pressure were identified. Data on all-cause mortality rates for only patients with diabetes mellitus at baseline were extracted from each study and are presented in Table 6–1.

If this was a *nonmeta-analysis systematic review article*, the conclusion would read:

"Six studies assessed long-term antihypertensive therapy in patients with diabetes mellitus and one showed a statistically significant reduction in all-cause mortality."

If this systematic review was a *meta-analysis*, the conclusion would read:

"Meta-analysis of the six studies (2302 patients) showed that all-cause mortality was reduced by antihypertensive medications in patients with diabetes mellitus (weighted mortality rate 11.4% versus 15.4%, $P < .02$)."

Note that weighting means that data from larger studies are given more "weight" in the analysis: basically, this is adjustment for sample size differences among the studies.

If the study was a meta-analysis that used *individual patient data* (often called a *pooled* or *individual patient data review*), the conclusion would read:

"1182 patients were allocated to active treatment and 1220 to placebo in the six studies. After adjustment for differences in baseline age, sex, severity of hypertension and diabetes, and duration of treatment, the active treatment group showed a decreased risk for all-cause mortality..."

Individual patient data meta-analyses are very effective and powerful, but require long-term and financial commitments from both the persons who are completing the

Table 6–1

All-Cause Mortality for Diabetic Patients with Hypertension Treated with Antihypertension Drugs

Trial	Patients	Mortality (Drug vs Placebo)	Direction	*P*-value
SAVE	492	19% vs 24%	Decrease	Not significant
SOLVD I	647	18% vs 24%	Decrease	Not significant
SOLVD II	633	43% vs 42%	Increase	Not significant
Austrian	36	43% vs 23%	Increase	Not significant
BHAT	465	9% vs 14%	Decrease	Not significant
Timolol	99	13% vs 33%	Decrease	$P < .02$

meta-analysis and the original investigators. The original investigators must supply the data in usable format for each patient. In the U.K., several large meta-analyses have been done by funding an investigator from each original trial to work with other investigators to complete the individual patient data meta-analysis. One of the best known groups of reviewers is the Collaborative Group on Hormonal Factors in Breast Cancer. They completed their study on oral contraceptives in 1996,[12] on hormone replacement therapy in 1997,[13] and on tamoxifen in 1998.[14] These meta-analyses are powerful, and provide valuable clinical evidence; indexers at NLM have not provided special indexing for effective retrieval for these individual patient data meta-analyses.

Statistics

Many of the statistics we introduced in previous chapters are also used to describe the results of systematic review articles. Usually the statistics and numbers are presented as *weighted, pooled, typical, summary estimate,* or *combined* results (for example, weighted absolute risk reduction, pooled number needed to treat, typical odds ratio, combined sensitivity and specificity, and summary estimate of the relative risk).

Step 5: Presentation of the Results

Systematic review articles include data and results in several formats. The raw data —the data taken from each study—are usually presented in table form. These tables are often accompanied by written descriptions of the similarities and differences among the studies. In addition, the formal combinations of data for meta-analyses are presented in another table form, with a graphic representation of the combined data and summary statistics. These tables are supplemented with written information. This tabular and graphic presentation of the raw and combined data is best represented using the tables from a meta-analysis by Insua et al.[15] This systematic review was done to measure the effects on mortality and morbidity of treating hypertension in the elderly. Some controversy existed around the need to start treating high blood pressure in anyone over the age of 60. Table 6–2 includes the data that were extracted from each of the nine studies that Insua et al. included in their systematic review. The studies are listed in the table in order of underlying disease severity, starting with the one with the least severity. Frequently the trials are listed in chronological order or based on some other clinical feature of the patients or the trials. Each trial has its own column, and each row represents a data element taken from each study. Visually, we can see that the trial elements for this systematic review, although not identical, are very similar. Statistical testing of these data showed that the trials were similar enough to combine into a meta-analysis. The table includes systolic and diastolic blood pressure at baseline for intervention and control groups; differences in change from baseline in systolic and diastolic blood pressure at 5 years; and total mortality rates. Similar tables were constructed for the other outcomes in the study: all-causes mortality and mortality from stroke and coronary heart disease.

Meta-analysis of the data for mortality from coronary heart disease is shown in Table 6–3. Seven of the nine trials measured mortality from coronary heart disease, and they are listed, this time in chronological order starting with the oldest. "T" refers to

Table 6–2
Hypertension Results

					Study (Reference)				
	ANBP (62)	SHEP (74)	HDFP (73)	MRC (72)	PPC (65)	EWPHE (63)	Sprackling and Colleagues (13)	VA (50)	STOP-H (25)
Severity ranking	1	2	3	4	5	6	7	Not ranked	Not ranked
Mean follow-up, y	3.4	4.5	5.0	5.8	4.4	4.7	4.0	3.8	2.1
Mean blood pressure at entry, *mm Hg*									
Treatment Group									
Systolic	166.3	170.5	170.9	184.5	196.7	183.0	190.1	165.1†	195.0
Diastolic	100.7	76.7	101.6	91.0	98.7	101.1	106.7	104.7†	102.0
Control Group									
Systolic	163.9	170.1	169.1	184.5	196.1	182.0	197.7	162.1†	195.0
Diastolic	100.9	76.4	100.9	90.5	98.0	101.0	108.5	103.6†	102.0
5-year follow up									
Difference in diastolic blood pressure (treatment group – control group), *mm Hg*	–6.7	–3.4	–5.1	–5.9	–11	–10	–7.8	–18.6	–10.0
Difference in systolic blood pressure (treatment group – control group), *mm Hg*	ND	–11.1	ND	–6.3	–18	–22	–18.4	ND	–27.0
Death rate, %									
Treatment group	2.4	9.0	12.7	13.8	14.4	32.5	80.7	ND	4.4
Control group	3.1	10.2	15.8	14.2	14.8	35.1	73.7	ND	7.7

*ANBP = Australian National Blood Pressure Study; EWPHE = European Working Party on High Blood Pressure in the Elderly; HDFP = Hypertension and Follow-up Program; MRC = Medical Research Council; ND = not determinable; PPC = Practice in Primary Care; SHEP = Systolic Hypertension in the Elderly; STOP-H = Swedish Trial in Old Patients with Hypertension; VA = Veterans Administration Cooperative Study on Antihypertensive Agents. ND = not determinable.

† = Refers to entire study population.

Reprinted with permission from the American College of Physicians—American Society of Internal Medicine. From Insua et al.[15]

Table 6–3

Results of Meta-Analysis of Mortality End Points

All Cause Mortality		T	C	Odds Ratio (Log Scale) Favors Treatment ——— Favors Control
STUDY				0.1 0.2 0.5 1 2 5 10
HDFP	1979	153/1202	178/1172	
ANBP	1981	7/293	9/289	
Sprackling	1981	48/60	44/60	
EWPHE	1985	135/416	149/424	
PPC	1986	60/419	69/465	
SHEP	1991	213/2365	242/2371	
STOP	1991	36/812	63/815	
MRC	1992	301/2183	315/2213	
TOTAL		953/7750	1069/7809	
ODDS RATIO				0.88 (0.80)–0.97) P = 0.0092

Test for Heterogeneity: $\chi^2_H = 13$, df = 7, 0.10 > P > 0.05

Stroke Mortality		T	C	
STUDY				
HDFP	1979	17/1202	31/1172	
ANBP	1981	1/293	1/289	
EWPHE	1985	21/416	31/424	
PPC	1986	4/419	15/465	
SHEP	1991	10/2365	14/2371	
STOP	1991	4/812	15/815	
MRC	1992	37/2183	42/2213	
TOTAL		94/7690	149/7749	
ODDS RATIO				0.64 (0.49)–0.82) P = 0.0005

Test for Heterogeneity: $\chi^2_H = 17.7$, df = 6, P < 0.01

CHD Mortality		T	C	
STUDY				
HDFP	1979	54/1202	68/1172	
ANBP	1981	1/293	4/289	
EWPHE	1985	29/416	47/424	
PPC	1986	25/419	28/465	
SHEP	1991	59/2365	73/2371	
STOP	1991	10/812	20/815	
MRC	1992	85/2183	110/2213	
TOTAL		263/7690	350/7749	
ODDS RATIO				0.75 (0.64)–0.88) P = 0.00055

Tests for Heterogeneity: $\chi^2_H = 40.3$, df = 6, P < 0.001

treatment group and "C" refers to the control group; and the columns here include the number of persons in each group in each trial, and how many had the outcome in question: in this case, coronary heart disease. The graphic presentation of each study under the column heading *Odds Ratio* gives the results of each study. For example, the first study is the HDFP study, and the OR represented by the "dot" shows that the outcome from the treatment favors the treatment group (treatment is better than no treatment); but the confidence interval *crosses* 1.0. This "crossing" means that the results are not statistically significant, and that only a trend towards decreased mortality from coronary heart disease was shown in the first trial.

The second trial shows similar results, except that, because so many fewer events occurred, the confidence intervals are wider (longer in the graphical representation); and again, because they cross 1.0, the results are not statistically significant. All seven trials favor the treatment group for treatment of hypertension to prevent coronary heart disease, but only one reaches statistical significance: and that one does so just barely. When, however, the results of the seven trials that measure coronary heart disease mortality are combined (graphically at the bottom of the table), and weighting is applied to the data from each trial to account for differences in numbers of persons in the trials, the final results are, on the contrary, highly statistically significant: mortality from coronary heart disease is reduced by treating hypertension in elderly persons (OR 0.75, 95% CI 0.64 to 0.88, $P = .00055$).

One other interesting item from this study is the final author, Tom Chalmers. He was a colorful and productive researcher, and one of his first studies was the famous unblinded trial of vitamin C that we referred to previously. Chalmers was also one of the first and foremost proponents of health care systematic reviews, and one of the founders of the Cochrane Collaboration. Systematic review articles and the New England Cochrane Center owe much to his leadership. Also of note is that his cottage in New England was used to film *On Golden Pond*. This cottage was the site of much work on the development of systematic review articles.

SUMMARY

Systematic reviews and meta-analyses tend to be prepared more carefully and concentrate more on collection and presentation of evidence than other review articles. The Evidence-Based Working Group[16] lists the features of systematic reviews in order of their clinical importance in their *Users' Guides*. They are a focused clinical question, explicit inclusion and exclusion criteria, strong retrieval methods that suggest that important, relevant studies were not missed, individual studies assessed reliably for validity, and that studies and their results were similar and shown to be similar.

There are three types of systematic review articles, and each requires its own retrieval process in MEDLINE. Systematic reviews that are not meta-analyses are indexed using the publication type REVIEW. To distinguish it from other nonsystematic review articles, the textwords MEDLINE, CINAHL, handsearch, and so on can be used as textwords ORed in with the REVIEW (publication type). Indexers have started to index for the study type also—for example, a systematic review article on a therapy topic will be indexed using clinical trials (MeSH) or randomized controlled trials (MeSH), whereas a diagnostic systematic review article would be indexed with sensitivity and specificity (MeSH); an etiology systematic review article would be indexed with case-control studies (MeSH), cohort studies (MeSH) or risk (MeSH); and a prognosis systematic review article would be indexed with cohort studies (MeSH).

Meta-analyses have both a MeSH and publication type to use in retrievals along with appropriate textwords—meta-analysis (publication type) or meta-analysis (MeSH) or meta-analysis (textword). Indexing for individual patient data meta-analyses has not been formalized, and retrieval is difficult, because most of these meta-analyses are indexed as original studies.

MEDLINE

Mesh and Textwords for Systematic Review Articles

Mesh
Meta-analysis
Grateful Medline
MEDLARS
    MEDLINE

Publication Type
Meta-analysis*

Textwords
Metaanaly:*
Meta-analy:*
Meta analy:*
Metanaly:
Systematic overview: or systematic review :
Quantitative overview: or quantitative review:
Methodologic: overview: or methodologic: review:
Collaborative: overview: or collaborative: review:
Integrative research review:
Research integration
Handsearch: or handsearch: or manual search:
Pooled data (careful not to get pooled blood, etc.)
Mantel haenszel
Peto
Dersimonian or der simonian
Fixed effect:

Electronic or bibliographic database:
MEDLINE (note MEDLINE as a textword retrieves review articles in which
    a MEDLINE search has been run to retrieve the articles for inclusion)
CINAHL
Psychinfo, psycinfo, psychlit, psyclit (make sure you use both correct and
    incorrect spellings)
Embase Excerpta medica
Medlars
Scisearch, Science Citation Index, isi citation databases, or web of science
Ovid, Winspirs, Blaise, BIDS, etc.

CINAHL Database of Nursing and Allied Health Literature

CINAHL Index Words, Document Types, and Textwords for Systematic Review Articles

Index Terms
Meta-analysis
Literature review
Literature searching
    Computerized literature searching
    Computerized literature searching, end user

CINAHL Document Types
Systematic review

Textwords
Use same as for MEDLINE except for the line "CINAHL" the search strategy should be:
Cinahl not (cinahl information.ab. or classification term.pt. or cinahl note.ab. or cinahl
    abstract.ab.)

CINAHL thesaurus terms selected by Katy Nesbit
All extracts from the CINAHL® Thesaurus Copyright © 1999, Cinahl Information Systems. Reprinted
with permission from Cinahl Information Systems.

PsycINFO

Index Words and Publication Types for Systematic Review Articles

Index Terms
Meta-analysis
Literature review

Publication Type or Form/Content Type
Meta analysis
Literature review—research review

Textwords
Use same list as for MEDLINE

PsycINFO terms selected by Jean Sullivant

EMBASE/EXCERPTA MEDICA

Index Terms, Links, and EMTAGS for Systematic Reviews

Index Terms
Meta-analysis
Review
Short survey

Links (subheadings)
(many could be listed—see listings in other chapters)

Emtags (publication types)
Review (has extensive bibiliography)
Survey (short piece with shorter bibliography)

Textwords
Use same list as for MEDLINE

MEDLINE HEDGES

No proved hedges exist for retrieving systematic reviews, meta-analyses, and individual patient meta-analyses. However, short and long search strategies have been developed with input from clinicians and librarians. The shorter one is published as part of a series on systematic review articles published in the *Annals of Internal Medicine* in 1997.[17] The longer one has been submitted for publication.

COMPREHENSIVE SEARCH STRATEGY FOR SYSTEMATIC REVIEWS: SHORT VERSION

001   meta-analysis (publication type)
002   meta-anal: (truncated textword)
003   metaanal: (truncated textword)
004   quantitative: review: or quantitative: overview: (truncated textwords)

005   systematic: review: or systematic: overview: (truncated textwords)
006   methodologic: review: or methodologic overview: (truncated textwords)
007   review (publication type) and medline (textword)
008   1 or 2 or 3 or 4 or 5 or 6 or 7

COMPREHENSIVE SEARCH STRATEGY FOR SYSTEMATIC REVIEWS: LONG VERSION

001   meta-analysis (publication type or MeSH)
002   (meta-anal: or metaanal:) (textword)
003   (quantitativ: review: or quantitativ: overview:) (textword)
004   (systematic: review: or systematic: overview:) (textword)
005   (methodologic: review: or methodologic: overview:) (textword)
006   (integrative research review: or research integration:) (textword)
007   quantitativ: synthes: (textword)
008   1 or 2 or 3 or 4 or 5 or 6 or 7
009   review: (publication type of MeSH) or review: (textword) or overview: (textword)
010   (medline or medlars) (textword or MeSH) or embase (textword)
011   (scisearch or psychinfo or psycinfo) (textword)
012   (psychlit or psyclit) (textword)
013   (hand search: or manual search:) (textword)
014   (electronic database: or bibliographic database:) (textword)
015   (pooling or pooled analys: or mantel haenszel) (textword)
016   (peto or der simonian or dersimonian or fixed effect:) (textword)
017   10 or 11 or 12 or 13 or 14 or 15 or 16
018   17 and 9
019   9 or 18

EXAMPLES

Example 6–1
Systematic review: therapy
Kearon C, Hirsh J. Starting prophylaxis for venous thromboembolism postoperatively. Arch Intern Med 1995;155:366–72.

This systematic review by Kearon et al. is on a topic that has clinical importance to many. People who have surgery are at an increased risk for venous thromboembolism (deep venous thrombosis or pulmonary embolism), either of which can be fatal. The venous thromboemboli, or blood clots, can be treated, but clinically it is better to prevent them before they form. The MEDLINE terms used in searching were: embolism, thrombosis, and prophylaxis; and personal reprint files, bibliographies of consensus papers, reviews, book chapters, and studies were checked. The inclusion criteria were:

MEDLINE Record for Example 6–1

Unique Identifier   95150742

Authors   Kearon C. Hirsh J.

Institution   McMaster University, Hamilton, Ontario.

Title   Starting prophylaxis for venous thromboembolism postoperatively [see comments]. [Review] [40 refs]

Source   Archives of Internal Medicine. 155(4):366–72, 1995 Feb 27.

MeSH Subject Headings
Clinical Trials
Human
Postoperative Care
*Postoperative Complications/pc [Prevention & Control]
Preoperative Care
Research Design
Support, Non-U.S. Gov't
Thromboembolism/et [Etiology]
*Thromboembolism/pc [Prevention & Control]

Abstract
A large proportion of hospitalized patients who are at high risk for venous thromboembolism (VTE) do not receive prophylaxis. Reluctance to use VTE prophylaxis in surgical patients may be due to fear of perioperative bleeding when anticoagulants are given preoperatively. We preformed a **literature review** to determine (1) whether prophylaxis for VTE is effective when it is started postoperatively and (2) the relative efficacy of preoperatively and postoperatively initiated prophylaxis. Studies were included in the review (1) if they were **randomized trials** with "blind" assessment of appropriate VTE outcomes, and (2) if prophylaxis was started postoperatively. Randomized, controlled trials establish that pharmacologic and nonpharmacologic methods of prophylaxis that are effective when started preoperatively are also effective when they are started postoperatively, with relative risks for VTE of 0.16 to 0.49. Low rates of VTE in noncontrolled randomized trials that included postoperatively initiated prophylactic regimens support this finding. The relative efficacy of preoperatively and postoperatively initiated VTE prophylaxis could not be determined definitively, as direct comparisons of the same regimens have not been performed. Indirect comparisons suggest that any loss of efficacy resulting from deferring VTE prophylaxis until after surgery is unlikely to be marked. Randomized trials are required to resolve this question. This comparison may be of greatest clinical importance when twice-daily, low-molecular-weight heparin is used to prevent VTE after major orthopedic surgery. [References: 40]

Publication Type   Journal Article. **Review.** Review, Tutorial.

- Single-blind or double-blind randomized controlled trials.
- Patients received prophylaxis after surgery or standard therapy, another method of prophylaxis, or prophylaxis before surgery.
- Timing of prophylaxis was clear.
- Venous thromboembolism (deep venous thrombosis and pulmonary embolism) was diagnosed without knowledge of treatment assignment.

Kearon et al. found 12 studies and one abstract that met these criteria. Data could not be combined because of differences across studies. (No meta-analyses were done.) Overall, postoperative prophylaxis was seen to be effective in almost all studies.

Retrieval Can Be Done Using Any of the Following:

Indexing	Clinical trials (MeSH)
	Review (publication type)
Textwords	Literature review (abstract)
	Randomized trials (abstract)

Example 6–2

Meta-analysis: diagnosis and screening (used for the development of a clinical practice guideline)

Carlson KJ, Skates SJ, Singer DE. Screening for ovarian cancer. Ann Intern Med 1994;121:124–32.

American College of Physicians. Screening for ovarian cancer; recommendations and rationale. Ann Intern Med 1994;121:141–2.

Carlson et al. completed this well-done meta-analysis for the American College of Physicians. An internal committee of the College used the data from it to develop clinical practice guidelines on screening women for ovarian cancer. Fourteen studies were identified and combined. For ultrasonography, the summary (combined) estimate of sensitivity was 85% (95% CI 80% to 90%) and of specificity was 94% (CI 93% to 94%). Their conclusion was that for women without a family history of ovarian cancer, screening is not recommended. Other women with risk factors, including a positive family history, must carefully make up their own minds on screening after weighing the alternative screening tests including no testing, and their implications.

Retrieval Can Use Any of the Following:

MeSH indexing	Review (publication type)
	Incidence
	Predictive value of tests
	Risk factors
	Sensitivity and specificity

Textwords	MEDLINE (abstract)
	Test operating characteristics (abstract)
	False-positive results (abstract)
	Meta-analysis (abstract)
	Risk factors (abstract)
	effectiveness (abstract)

Example 6–3
Meta-analysis using individual patient data: etiology

Cholesterol, diastolic blood pressure, and stroke: 13,000 strokes in 450,000 people in 45 prospective cohorts. Prospective studies collaboration. Lancet 1995;346:1647–53.

Funding for this study was provided by Merch, Sharp, and Dohm and the U.K. Medical Research Council to determine if an association exists between total blood cholesterol levels and stroke. Forty-five cohort studies with 448, 415 patients for 15-to-30 year follow-up were included in this meta-analysis. Because it collected and analyzed data from each patient, it was an individual patient data meta-analysis. Thirteen thousand three hundred and ninety-seven patients had a stroke during follow-up. Results of the meta-analysis showed that stroke was not associated with cholesterol levels. Diastolic blood pressure was, however, associated with stroke, with an adjusted relative risk for stroke of 1.84 for every 10 mm Hg increase in diastolic blood pressure (95% CI 1.80 to 1.90).

MEDLINE Record for Example 6–2

Unique Identifier   94288379

Authors   Anonymous.

Title   Screening for ovarian cancer: recommendations and rationale. American College of Physicians [see comments].

Source   Annals of Internal Medicine. 121(2):141–2, 1994 Jul 15.

MeSH Subject Headings
    Female
    Human
    *Mass Screening/st [Standards]
    *Ovarian Neoplasms/pc [Prevention & Control]
    United States

Publication Type   Guideline. Journal Article. Practice Guideline

MEDLINE Record for Example 6–2 continued

Unique Identifier   94288377

Authors   Carlson KJ. Skates SJ. Singer DE.

Institution   Massachusetts General Hospital, Boston.

Title   Screening for ovarian cancer [see comments]. [Review] [83 refs]

Source   Annals of Internal Medicine. 121(2):124–32, 1994 Jul 15.

MeSH Subject Headings
Antigens, Tumor-Associated, Carbohydrate/bl [Blood]
Female
Human
Incidence
Mass Screening/mt [Methods]
*Mass Screening
Ovarian Neoplasms/ep [Epidemiology]
Ovarian Neoplasms/im [Immunology]
*Ovarian Neoplasms/pc [Prevention & Control]
Ovarian Neoplasms/us [Ultrasonography]
Predictive Value of Tests
Risk Factors
Sensitivity and Specificity
Support, Non-U.S. Gov't
United States/ep [Epidemiology]

Abstract
PURPOSE: To critically review the available evidence for screening asymptomatic women for ovarian cancer with ultrasonography or the CA 125 radioimmunoassay (CA 125) or both. DATA SOURCES: A **MEDLINE** search of the English-language literature and bibliographies of published studies providing estimates of ovarian cancer risk and **test operating characteristics** (based on observational studies and **meta-analyses**) and **effectiveness** of treatment according to stage of disease (based on randomized trials). Published mathematical models simulating screening for ovarian cancer in specific populations were also included. Death from ovarian cancer and morbidity from surgical procedures were the principal outcomes considered. RESULTS: Age and family history are the most important **risk factors** for ovarian cancer. Annual screening with CA 125 or ultrasound in women older than 50 years without a family history of ovarian cancer would result in more than 30 **false-positive results** for every ovarian cancer detected. False-positive tests are likely to require invasive testing, often including laparotomy. There is currently no direct evidence that mortality from ovarian cancer would be decreased by screening. CONCLUSIONS: Available evidence does not support either screening of pre- or postmenopausal women without a family history of ovarian cancer or routine screening in women with a family history of ovarian cancer in one or more relatives (without evidence of a hereditary cancer syndrome). Women from a family with the rare hereditary ovarian cancer syndrome are at high risk for the disease and should be referred to a gynecologic oncologist. [References: 83]

Publication Type   Journal Article. **Review.** Review, Multicase. Review, Tutorial.

MEDLINE Record for Example 6–3

Unique Identifier   96110598

Authors   Anonymous.

Institution   Cholesterol, diastolic blood pressure, and stroke: 13,000 strokes in 450,000 people in 45 prospective cohorts. Prospective studies collaboration [see comments].

Source   Lancet. 346(8991–8992):1647–53, 1995 Dec 23–30.

MeSH Subject Headings
Age Factors	Female
Aged	Human
*Blood Pressure	Male
Cerebrovascular Disorders/bl [Blood]	Middle Age
*Cerebrovascular Disorders/ep [Epidemiology]	Mongoloid Race
Cerebrovascular Disorders/pp [Physiopathology]	**Prospective Studies**
*Cholesterol/bl [Blood]	**Risk Factors**
Cohort Studies	Support, Non-U.S. Gov't
Coronary Disease/co [Complications]	

Abstract
Individual studies of stroke have not clearly answered two questions: on the relation, if any, between total blood cholesterol and stroke; and on how the strength of the relation between diastolic blood pressure and stroke varies with age. The associations of blood cholesterol and diastolic blood pressure with subsequent stroke rates were investigated by review of 45 prospective observational **cohorts** involving 450,000 individuals with 5–30 years of follow-up (mean 16 years, total 7.3 million person-years of observation), during which 13,397 participants were recorded as having had a stroke. Most of these were fatal strokes in studies that recorded only **mortality** and not **incidence**, but about one-quarter were from studies that recorded both fatal and non-fatal strokes. After standardization for age, there was no association between blood cholesterol and stroke except, perhaps, in those under 45 years of age when screened. This lack of association was not influenced by adjustment for sex, diastolic blood pressure, history of coronary disease, or ethnicity (Asian or non-Asian). However, because the types of the strokes were not centrally available, the lack of any overall relation might conceal a positive association with ischaemic stroke together with a negative association with haemorrhagic stroke. When the highest and the lowest of the six blood pressure categories were compared, the difference in usual diastolic blood pressure was 27 mm Hg (102 vs 75 mm Hg), and there was a fivefold difference in stroke risk. This fivefold difference was seen both in those with a pre-existing history of coronary heart disease and in those without it. The proportional difference in stroke **risk**, however, was more extreme in middle than in old age. Among those aged < 45, 45–64, and 65+ when screened, the differences in the **relative risks** of stroke (between the highest diastolic blood pressure category and a combination of the lowest two categories) were tenfold, fivefold, and twofold, respectively. However, because the absolute stroke risks are greater in old age, the absolute differences in the annual stroke rates showed an opposite pattern, being 2, 5, and 8 per thousand, respectively. This suggests that the effects of therapeutic blood pressure reductions should be assessed separately in middle age and in old age.

Publication Type   Journal Article.

Retrieval Can Use Any of the Following:

MeSH indexing	Age factors
	Cohort studies
	Prospective studies
	Risk factors
	Note: *no indexing for systematic review articles or meta-analysis*—this individual patient data systematic review article is almost impossible to retrieve, as are almost all individual patient data meta-analyses!
Textwords	Cohorts (abstract)
	Risk (abstract)
	Relative risks
	Mortality (abstract)
	Incidence (abstract)

Example 6–4
Systematic review: prognosis
Bucher HC. Social support and prognosis following first myocardial infarction. J Gen Intern Med 1994;9:409–17(no abstract available).

Bucher wanted to examine the contributions of psychosocial factors, especially social support, to the prognosis of patients after a first myocardial infarction. Nine cohort studies (11,675 patients) and two randomized, controlled trials (818 patients) were included in this nonmeta-analysis systematic review. Four of seven studies that measured social support were associated with an increasing risk for cardiac death. The biggest risk factor across all of the studies for all patients after a myocardial infarction was lack of a spouse or close confidant (OR for death from one study 3.4, 95% CI 1.84 to 6.20).

Retrieval Can Use Any of the Following:

MeSH indexing	Review (publication type)
	Prognosis
	Risk assessment
Textwords	(Note the article has no abstract, and the title says nothing that can be used for intelligent retrieval: this valuable study is lost to retrieval.)

MEDLINE Record for Example 6–4

Unique Identifier   95017185

Authors   Bucher HC.

Institution   Medizinische Universitats-Poliklinik, Kantonsspital Basel, Switzerland.

Title   Social support and prognosis following first myocardial infarction [see comments]. [Review] [106 refs]

Source   Journal of General Internal Medicine. 9(7):409–17, 1994 Jul.

MeSH Subject Headings
Female
Human
Male
Myocardial Infarction/mo [Mortality]
Myocardial Infarction/pc [Prevention & Control]
*Myocardial Infarction/pp [Physiopathology]
*Myocardial Infarction/px [Psychology]
Prognosis
Recurrence
Risk Assessment
*Social Support

Publication Type   Journal Article. **Review.** Review, Academic.

Example 6–5
Systematic review: economics
Keanan SP, Massel D, Inman KJ, Sibbald WJ. A systematic review of the cost-effective-ness of noncardiac transitional care units. Chest 1998;113:172–7.

This study was done to summarize the available data on the cost-effectiveness of non-cardiac transition care units. The MEDLINE search strategy included the search terms *intermediate care unit, respiratory care unit,* and *step-down unit.* Bibliographies of review articles and studies were checked as were personal files. Although all studies claimed that their noncardiac care unit was cost-effective, all studies included design flaws that were serious enough to undermine the validity of the individual conclusions. In addition, the studies were so varied that meta-analysis could not be done to combine the data.

Retrieval Can Be Done Using Any of the Following:

MeSH indexing	Cost-benefit analysis
	MEDLINE
	Retrospective studies
	(Note no indexing for review or meta-analysis)
Textwords	Systematic review (title)
	Critically appraise (abstract)
	Computerized literature search (abstract)
	MEDLINE (abstract)
	Current Contents (abstract)
	HealthSTAR (abstract)
	Bibliographies (abstract)
	Personal files (abstract)
	Data synthesis (abstract)
	Data extraction (abstract)

Example 6–6
Systematic review: qualitative studies
Paterson BL, Thorne S, Dewis M. Adapting to and managing diabetes. Image J Nurs Sch 1998;30:57–62.

Quantitative studies provide firm, precise estimates of population means across groups of patients (for example, the rate of myocardial infarction at 5 years in adults with high cholesterol levels who took gemfibrozil was 2.3%). Qualitative studies provide an alter-native method of assessing patients and health issues. Qualitative studies provide rich, broad-based understanding of their experiences and understanding of their health care in the context of disease, conditions, or situations (see Chapter 10). Researchers who produce qualitative studies usually work intensely over a long period of time with a

MEDLINE Record for Example 6–5

Unique Identifier   98101536

Authors   Keenan SP. Massel D. Inman KJ. Sibbald WJ.

Institution   Richard Ivey Critical Care Trauma Center, Victoria Campus, University of Western Ontario, London, Canada.

Title   A **systematic review** of the cost-effectiveness of noncardiac transitional care units.

Source   Chest. 113(1):172–7, 1998 Jan.

MeSH Subject Headings
Cost-Benefit Analysis
Data Interpretation, Statistical
*Health Care Costs
Health Services Research/mt [Methods]
Human
*Intermediate Care Facilities/ec [Economics]
Intermediate Care Facilities/sn [Statistics & Numerical Data]
MEDLINE
Reproducibility of Results
Retrospective Studies
Support, Non-U.S. Gov't
United States

Abstract
OBJECTIVE: To **critically appraise** and summarize the studies examining the cost-effectiveness of noncardiac transitional care units (TCUs). DATA SOURCES: We conducted a **computerized literature search** using **MEDLINE**, and **Current Contents** from January 1, 1986 to December 31, 1995 and **HealthSTAR** from January 1, 1989 to December 31, 1995 with the key words intermediate care unit, respiratory care unit, and step-down unit. **Bibliographies** of all selected articles and review articles were examined. **Personal files** were also reviewed. STUDY SELECTION: (1) Population: patients in a noncardiac TCU of an acute-care institution; (2) intervention: addition of a noncardiac TCU to the institution; and (3) outcomes: patient outcome-survival and associated costs. DATA EXTRACTION: The necessary data were abstracted and study validity was evaluated by two independent reviewers using a modification of previously published criteria. DATA SYNTHESIS: The studies were summarized qualitatively; upon inspection, they were too heterogeneous to allow quantitative analysis. While the studies all claimed that their TCUs were cost-effective, the economic evaluation designs were flawed to such an extent that the validity of the conclusions is suspect. CONCLUSIONS: To date, the evidence in the literature is insufficient to determine under which circumstances, if any, TCUs are a cost-effective alternative technology to the traditional institution with only ICU and general ward beds.

Publication Type   Journal Article.

small number of patients, either individually or in small groups. Qualitative studies can also be combined in systematic reviews. This systematic review by Paterson et al. was done to expand the understanding of the lived experience described by people with diabetes mellitus. Forty-three qualitative studies were identified from six computerized databases. "Meta-ethnography" was applied, and the conclusion is that learning how to balance living and the disease process is a developmental process in which one learns how to assume control of diabetes management.

Retrieval Can Use Any of the Following:

MeSH indexing	Meta-analysis (publication type)
Textwords	Meta-analysis (abstract)
	Meta-ethnography (abstract)
	Computerized data bases (abstract)

ASSIGNMENT

Try these questions out in MEDLINE, HealthStar, and any other database you like.

1. You never really believed in chiropractors until your lower back "went out" in the past year. What do systematic review articles say about chronic low-back pain, and how do the chiropractors fare in these assessments?
2. Depression in hospitalized patients is starting to be taken seriously as a risk factor for death and slower rehabilitation. Have any systematic review articles been done that assess depression in patients who have had a stroke or myocardial infarction?
3. Case managers make intuitive sense for increasing the effectiveness of inpatient treatment and complete and timely discharge planning. Has anyone pulled this information together in one place in a systematic review?
4. Fish oil is purported to be good for persons with rheumatoid arthritis. What does the meta-analysis literature say specifically regarding its effects? (*Hint*: fish oil has many, many names.)

FURTHER READING

In 1997, the *Annals of Internal Medicine* produced a series of articles on systematic review articles for clinicians. It provides a good background on the topic in a readable format. The citations are listed in the *Further Reading* section at the end of this book.

MEDLINE Record for Example 6–6

Unique Identifier   98211113

Authors   Paterson BL. Thorne S. Dewis M.

Institution   School of Nursing, University of British Columbia, Vancouver, Canada. feenstra:ccco.net

Title   Adapting to and managing diabetes.

Source   Image — the Journal of Nursing Scholarship. 30(1):57–62, 1998.

MeSH Subject Headings
Decision Making
Diabetes Mellitus/nu [Nursing]
*Diabetes Mellitus/rh [Rehabilitation]
Human
Internal-External Control
Motivation
*Self Care
Support, Non-U.S. Gov't

Abstract
PURPOSE: To advance understanding of the lived experience of diabetes as described in published research and theses. **Meta-analysis** extends the analysis of individual research studies beyond individual experience to incorporate dominant system beliefs and health system ideologies. ORGANIZING FRAMEWORK: Curtin and Lubkin's (1990) conceptualization of the experience of chronic illness. SOURCES: Forty-three qualitative interpretive research reports in six **computerized data bases** 1980–1996 pertaining to the lived experience of diabetes and published in nursing, in the social sciences, and in allied health journals were used. METHODS: **Meta-ethnography** in which trustworthiness was achieved by using multiple researchers, identifying negative or disconfirming cases, and testing rival hypotheses. FINDINGS: Balance is the determinant metaphor of the experience of diabetes. People learn to balance diabetes through their experience and experimentation with strategies for managing their illness. CONCLUSIONS: Learning to balance is a developmental process in which one learns to assume control of diabetes management. Support for such development requires that nurses know their clients as individuals and value the expertise they have gained in living with diabetes. Control of blood sugar levels within a prescribed range may be a goal established by professionals, but the goal of healthy balance determines a person's willingness to assume an active role in self-care.

Publication Type   Journal Article. **Meta-Analysis.**

COCHRANE COLLABORATION

In an influential book published more than 25 years ago, Archie Cochrane, a British obstetrician, drew attention to the fact that health care professionals were not using evidence from the wealth of randomized controlled trials that was available to them. He is quoted:[18]

> "It is surely a great criticism of our profession that we have not organized a critical summary, by speciality or subspeciality, adapted periodically of all relevant randomized controlled trials."

The Cochrane Collaboration has developed to meet this challenge. The Collaboration is a worldwide network of health professionals, librarians, lay persons, and patients who work together to identify, collect, and synthesize the knowledge from randomized controlled trials and to prepare and maintain systematic reviews. The international endeavor aims to ensure that eventually all areas of health care that have been evaluated using randomized controlled trials will be covered using systematic review methods and made available to anyone who makes, or helps to make, patient care decisions. All areas of health care are included, and a strong lay component has been built in from the start.

The Cochrane Collaboration started with a group of obstetricians and neonatologists who undertook to collect and evaluate all randomized controlled trials in perinatal medicine (defined as from conception through to age 1 month). Two books were produced.[19,20] Each chapter was a systematic review. Besides print form, the chapters were also made available on computer as the *Oxford Database of Perinatal Trials*. In addition, the authors of each chapter were committed to keeping the database and text up-to-date as new relevant studies were published.

The books became valuable tools for many health care providers who worked with pregnant women and newborn infants. Archie Cochrane praised the work as "a real milestone in the history of randomized controlled trials and in the evaluation of care." He also suggested that this model be expanded to cover all areas of health and health care.[21] His peers took up the challenge after his death.

Participation in the Cochrane Collaboration is on a voluntary basis and each person has affiliations to a national center and belongs to a content-based review group, such as stroke or musculoskeletal disorders. Each review group is responsible for helping collect randomized controlled trials in their area of expertise. This often involves hand searching specialty and national journals and conference proceedings in addition to usual literature search methods. Review groups also produce and maintain systematic reviews in areas of relevance to the group. These collections of randomized controlled trials and systematic reviews are published as part of the *Cochrane Library*.

THE COCHRANE LIBRARY

The Cochrane Library is a computerized version on the Internet and in CD-ROM format of Cochrane's dream in action. It has six major parts. Of greatest importance is a collection all of the systematic reviews developed and maintained by the Collaboration.

Approximately 900 of these systematic reviews are now available, and they cover a broad range of important topics. In addition to the completed systematic reviews, protocols are also included describing work in progress. This allows others interested in the topic the benefit of work to date, and also allows for input into the final review. Second, the *Library* includes a collection of more than 1800 citations (with abstracts) to other systematic reviews. These abstracts are author-generated abstracts or custom-written abstracts produced by the National Health Services Centre for Reviews and Dissemination at the University of York in the U.K. Technical reports and technology assessments are included. Third, the *Library* contains citations to over 200,000 randomized and pseudorandomized controlled trials in all languages dating back to the late 1880s. This segment of the *Library* is growing rapidly. The Cochrane Collaboration works closely with the National Library of Medicine to ensure indexing quality and consistency. Any use of the term *controlled clinical trial (publication type)* is an indication that the Collaboration has worked with the National Library of Medicine to perfect the indexing of that article. Studies indexed as controlled clinical trials were identified by members of the Cochrane Collaboration, and they are retrospectively reindexed by MEDLINE and HealthStar indexers. The fourth part of the *Cochrane Library* is a database of citations and abstracts of methodology papers related to the Collaboration and systematic review methods. The *Cochrane Handbook* is also part of the *Library*, and is also available at *http://Mcmaster.hiru.ca/cochrane/handbook/default.htm*. It includes many useful chapters on methodologies and techniques for producing systematic reviews and administrative features and procedures for sites and groups. It has some wonderful search strategies for capturing all clinical trials in many databases. The last section has contact and other related information about the collaboration itself. Many other projects are underway by the various Cochrane groups, national centers, and annual meeting planners, and more information can be found at various Internet sites, such as *http://hiru.mcmaster.ca/cochrane/overview.htm*. Update Software, the producers of the *Cochrane Library*, provide free access to the abstracts of all the systematic reviews in the *Cochrane Library*. Their URL is: *http://hiru.mcmaster.ca/cochrane/revabstr/abidx.htm*. In addition CINAHL now indexes the Cochrane systematic reviews.

GEOGRAPHIC SITES

The 14 Cochrane Centers (geographic sites) are:
Australasian Cochrane Centre
Brazilian Cochrane Centre
Canadian Cochrane Centre
Dutch Cochrane Centre
French Cochrane Centre
German Cochrane Center
Italian Cochrane Centre
New England Cochrane Center
Nordic Cochrane Centre

San Antonio Cochrane Center
San Francisco Cochrane Center
South African Cochrane Centre
Spanish Cochrane Center
U.K. Cochrane Centre

SEARCHING THE LIBRARY

The *Cochrane Library*, which is updated quarterly, has grown to a size where it is now a formidable clinical and research tool. The systematic reviews cover many important topics for health care professionals and administrators. Consider trying it out for your next health care question needs. Also go back to the last set of search exercises, and try the questions using the *Cochrane Library*.

REFERENCES

1. Tryba M. Prophylaxis of stress ulcer bleeding. A meta-analysis. J Clin Gastroenterol 1991;13 Suppl 2:S44–55.
2. Hatala R, Dinh T, Cook DJ. Once-daily aminoglycoside dosing in immunocompetent adults: a meta-analysis. Ann Intern Med 1996;124:717–25.
3. Pearson K. Report on certain enteric fever inoculation statistics. Br Med J 1904;3:1243–6.
4. Goldberger J. Typhoid bacillus carriers. Bull Hyg Lab 1907;35:165–74.
5. Glass GV, McGaw B, Smith ML. Meta-analysis in social research. Beverly Hills: Sage Publications; 1981.
6. Pauling L. The significance of evidence about ascorbic acid and the common cold. Proc Natl Acad Sci U S A 1971;68:2678–81.
7. Macharia WM, Leon G, Rowe BH, et al. An overview of interventions to improve compliance with appointment keeping for medical services. JAMA 1992;267:1813–7.
8. Wattenberg LW. An overview of chemoprevention: current status and future prospects. Proc Soc Exp Biol Med 1997;216:133–41.
9. Frick MH, Elo O, Haapa K, et al. Helsinki Heart Study: primary prevention trial with gemfibrozil in middle-aged men with dyslipidemia. N Engl J Med 1987;317:1237–45.
10. Schneider LS, Olin JT. Overview of clinical trials of hydergine in dementia. Arch Neurol 1994; 51:787–98.
11. Hoffman MA, Amiral J, Kohl B, et al. Hyperchomocyst(e)inemia and endothelial dysfunction in IDDM. Diabetes Care 1997;20:1880–6.
12. Collaborative Group on Hormonal Factors in Breast Cancer. Breast cancer and hormonal contraceptives: collaborative reanalysis of individual data on 53,297 women with breast cancer and 100, 239 women without breast cancer from 54 epidemiological studies. Lancet 1996;347: 1713–27.
13. Collaborative Group on Hormonal Factors in Breast Cancer. Breast cancer and hormone replacement therapy: collaborative reanalysis of data from 51 epidemiological studies of 52,705 women with breast cancer and 108,411 women without breast cancer. Lancet 1997;350: 1047–59.
14. Collaborative Group on Hormonal Factors in Breast Cancer. Tamoxifen for early breast cancer: an overview of the randomised trials. Lancet 1998;351:1451–67.
15. Insua JT, Sacks HS, Lau TS, et al. Drug treatment of hypertension in the elderly: a meta-analysis. Ann Intern Med 1994;121:355–62.

16. Oxman AD, Cook DL, Guyatt GH for the Evidence-Based Medicine Working Group. Users' guides to the medical literature. VI. How to use an overview. JAMA 1994;272:1367–71.

17. Hunt DL, McKibbon KA. Locating and appraising systematic reviews. Ann Intern Med 1997; 126:532–8.

18. Cochrane AL. Effectiveness and efficacy. Random reflections on health services. London: Nuffield Provincial Hospitals Trust; 1972. (Reprinted in 1989 in association with the BMJ.)

19. Chalmers I, Enkin M, Keirse MJNC, editors. Effective care in pregnancy and childbirth. Oxford: Oxford University Press; 1989.

20. Sinclair JC, Bracken MB, editors. Effective care of the newborn infant. Oxford: Oxford University Press; 1992.

21. Cochrane AL. Foreword. In: Chalmers I, Enkin M, Keirse MJNC, editors. Effective care in pregnancy and childbirth. Oxford: Oxford University Press; 1989.

Secondary Publications: Clinical Practice Guidelines

Practice guidelines are "systematically developed statements to assist practitioner and patient decisions about appropriate health care for specific clinical circumstances."[1] This definition was adopted by the U.S. Institute of Medicine Committee to Advise the Public Health Service on Practice Guidelines. Guidelines are produced by associations, foundations, or other clinical groups, and may be disseminated to group members, issued by government departments, or published in the journal literature. Guidelines range in size from a "care map" developed by the staff of a hospital intensive care unit to help guide and guarantee continuity of care for patients with acute stroke during their first week in the hospital to large, broadly based guidelines on topics such as incontinence or pressure sores. Estimates of the number of guidelines varies. In the U.S., national estimates range from 1600[2] to more than 26,000[3] that are available to health professionals.

CLINICAL EXAMPLE

The clinical example for this chapter is one developed by a committee of the Canadian Task Force on the Periodic Health Examination,[4] chaired by Dr. Elaine Wang. The committee was given responsibility to produce Canadian national guidelines to help health professionals encourage and promote breastfeeding. The 13-member committee included experts in family medicine, pediatrics, psychiatry, and epidemiology. They met two to three times a year for several years and used evidence from MEDLINE searches, bibliographies of relevant studies, and their clinical experience to make recommendations. Their guideline had two strong recommendations: to counsel and encourage women to choose breastfeeding for their infants; and to implement programs that would promote breastfeeding. After development, the recommendations were sent for peer review, re-examined, compared with other related national and international guidelines on breastfeeding, and then published and disseminated.

Guidelines are currently being promoted as a means for improving the quality of health care; optimizing patient outcomes; discouraging the use of ineffective or harmful interventions; improving and guaranteeing the consistency of care; identifying gaps in evidence; and helping balance costs and outcomes. Medical organizations, health services researchers, sponsors of health benefit plans, and public officials have expressed interest in their development and implementation. With the increased attention have come concerns about guidelines. Opinions are strong, both for and against the guidelines. For example, a Canadian survey of physician knowledge, attitudes, and use of guidelines was done:[5] one comment from a concerned physician was, "Guidelines are developed simply to control costs. They should be banned in perpetuity and those who promote them should be banished to the deepest pits of hell." Not everyone feels that strongly, but almost everyone has some feelings.

To address some of these concerns, questions have been raised on standardization and perfection of the specific methods used to develop guidelines; their clinical and methodological reliability; their validity; whether clinicians will interpret and apply them consistently under similar clinical circumstances; and whether, if applied properly, the guidelines will lead to the predicted health outcomes. To answer these questions, several groups are in the process of bringing order and quality to development of guidelines and evaluating their impact. The Canadian Task Force on the Periodic Health Examination and the U.S. Preventive Services Task Force are national organizations of health care professionals who have developed large collections of well-done, evidence-based guidelines for their respective countries. Their publications[6,7] each include almost 100 guidelines. The books provide comprehensive assistance for primary health care practitioners and others who deal with routine care. The organizations have worked together and shared expertise and evidence resources; the resulting guidelines, although similar, reflect national and regional differences. In addition, the U.S. Congress has assigned the Agency on Health Care Policy and Research (AHCPR) responsibility for determining the definitions and attributes of practice guidelines and their evaluation.[8]

EVIDENCE-BASED PRACTICE CENTERS

The AHCPR has designated 12 Evidence-Based Practice Centers to assemble the evidence for production of directed clinical practice guidelines.[9] Under contract, each center works with organizations that have requested AHCPR to produce a specific guideline. For example, McMaster University worked with the American Academy of Pediatricians and the American Psychiatric Association to produce a summary of the evidence for a guideline on the treatment of attention deficit-hyperactivity disorder in children and adults. Each center was assigned their first topic in late 1997, and a full report on each topic was completed in mid-1998.

Steps in the Production of a Clinical Practice Guideline

Good guidelines are produced using a six-step process:

1. Definition of the topic or process, including the target condition, interventions, patient population, clinical settings to be included, type of scientific evidence to be considered, and outcome measures to assess effectiveness and safety.

2. Assessment of clinical benefits and harms that includes review of scientific evidence (literature retrieval; evaluation of individual studies; including grading of the quality of the evidence and abstraction of the results; and synthesis of the evidence) and consideration of expert opinion.
3. Consideration of resource and feasibility issues.
4. Development of recommendations, including strength of the recommendations and the extent to which they are supported by scientific evidence.
5. Writing the guideline.
6. External review of the evidence and recommendations, and consideration of the clinical implications and adoption by the relevant health care community.

Evidence-based guidelines are based on levels of evidence: the stronger the evidence, the more faith a reader can put in the recommendation of the guideline. Recommendations are the "meat" of any guideline. They should be precise statements of specific actions to be taken or not taken in specific circumstances, and reflect the evidential strength for making that statement (for example, aspirin is not recommended for pregnant women with hypertension to prevent pre-eclampsia. Randomized controlled trials of aspirin have not shown any benefits for maternal or child mortality or morbidity.) Heffner[10] discusses further how EBHC helps with the development of clinical practice guidelines. Each group of guideline developers sets their own levels of strength of evidence. The Canadian Hypertension Society Consensus Development Conference has set the levels of evidence that follow.[11] Most guideline developers use a similar, but not identical, ranking of evidence.

Levels of Evidence for Rating Studies of Therapy, Prevention, and Quality Improvement

I. A randomized, controlled trial (RCT) that demonstrates a statistically significant difference in at least one important outcome—for example, survival or major illness; *or*, if the difference is not statistically significant, a RCT of adequate sample size to exclude a 25% difference in relative risk with 80% power, given the observed results.

II. A RCT that does not meet level I criteria.

III. A nonrandomized trial with contemporaneous controls selected by some systematic method (that is, not selected by perceived suitability for one of the treatment options for individual patients); *or* subgroup analysis of a RCT.

IV. A before and after study or case series (of at least 10 patients) with historical controls or controls drawn from other studies.

V. Case series (at least 10 patients) without controls.

VI. Case report (fewer than 10 patients).

Levels of Evidence for Rating Studies of Diagnosis

I. (a) Independent interpretation of test procedure (without knowledge of result of diagnostic standard).

(b) Independent interpretation of diagnostic standard (without knowledge of test procedure).

(c) Selection of patients or subjects who are suspected, but not known, to have the disorder of interest.

(d) Reproducible description of both the test and diagnostic standard.

(e) At least 50 patients with, and 50 without the disorder.

II. Meets four of the criteria in I.

III. Meets three of the criteria in I.

IV. Meets two of the criteria in I.

V. Meets one of the criteria in I.

VI. Meets none of the criteria in I.

Levels of Evidence for Rating Studies of Prognosis

I.   (a) Inception cohort.

(b) Reproducible inclusion and exclusion criteria.

(c) Follow-up of at least 80% of subjects.

(d) Statistical adjustment for extraneous prognostic factors (confounders).

(e) Reproducible description of outcome measures.

II. Inception cohort, but meets only three of the other criteria.

III. Inception cohort, but meets only two of the other criteria.

IV. Inception cohort, but meets only one of the other criteria.

V. Inception cohort, but meets none of the other criteria.

VI. Meets none of the criteria.

Levels of Evidence for Rating Review Articles

I.   (a) Comprehensive search for evidence.

(b) Avoidance of bias in selection of articles.

(c) Assessment of the validity of each cited article.

(d) Conclusions supported by the data and analysis presented.

II. Meets only three of the criteria in I.

III. Meets only two of the criteria in I.

IV. Meets only one of the criteria in I.

V. Meets none of the criteria in I.

Grading System for Recommendations

Each recommendation is also given a "grade" in addition to an assessment of the level or quality of the evidence. Again, these grades differ from group to group. The grades for the Canadian Hypertension are as follows:

A.   The recommendation is based on one or more studies at level I.

B.   The best evidence was at level II.

C.   The best evidence was at level III.
D.   The best evidence was lower than level III, and included expert opinion.

Another set of gradings for recommendations is the one used by the Canadian Task Force on the Periodic Health Examination and the U.S. Preventive Services Task Force for their recommendations:

A.   Strong evidence to support the recommendation.
B.   Weak evidence to support the recommendation.
C.   No evidence to support or refute the recommendation.
D.   Weak evidence to refute the recommendation.
E.   Strong evidence to refute the recommendation.

Two examples of recommendations from the Canadian Task Force show these gradings and levels:[12]

1.   "Fair evidence exists to include colonoscopy for the periodic health examination of patients in kindreds with cancer family syndrome (III, B)."
2.   "Insufficient evidence exists to include or exclude multiphasic screening in the periodic health examination of patients > 40 years old if they have no family history of colorectal cancer (I, C)."

ALTERNATIVE NAMES

The following 110 names are some, but not all, of the ones that have been used to refer to clinical guidelines. They are from a published MEDLINE search strategy produced by the British Columbia Office of Health Technology Assessment Centre for Health Services and Policy Research[13] and they can be used for retrieval in any search system.

clinical protocols
clinical or medical guidelines
clinical or medical standards
clinical or medical protocol
clinical or medical recommend:*
clinical or medical statement:
clinical or medical criteri:
clinical or medical polic:
clinical or medical option:
clinical or medical intervention:
practice or practise or care guideline:
practice or practise or care standard:
practice or practise or care protocol:
practice or practise or care recommend:
practice or practise or care statement:
practice or practise or care criteri:

practice or practise or care parameter:
practice or practise or care polic:
practice or practise or care option:
practice or practise or care intervention:
position paper or statement
health guideline
health planning guideline
flowchart:
consensus development conference:
physician's practice patterns or physicians' practice patterns
practice or practise pattern
medical or clinical necessity:
medical or clinical indicator:
reference standard
treatment guideline, standard, or protocol
treatment parameter or polic:
treatment option: or intervention:
prefer: practice or practise or treat:
planning guideline: or standard: or protocol:
planning recommend: or statement: or criteri:
performance guideline or standard: or protocol:
performance recommend: or statement: or criteri:
planning or performance parameter:
appropriate evaluat: or care
guideline: or standard: or protocol: and criteri:
medical or clinical review and criteri:
practice or practise review and criteri:
medical or clinical review:
practice or practise review:
management or care or performance review and criteri:
performance measure:
clinical or critical pathway
care map:
algorithm:
consensus develop conference:
practice guideline:

*the ":" means truncation—it will retrieve multiple endings on search words (for example, map: will retrieve map, maps, mapping, mapped, and also maple).

STRUCTURED ABSTRACTS FOR CLINICAL PRACTICE GUIDELINES

Just as the health care community has moved to implement more informative abstracts of clinical studies, a proposed structure for abstracts of clinical guidelines has been developed and implemented.[15] The section headings include:

- Objective.
- Option.
- Outcomes.
- Evidence.
- Values.
- Benefits, Harms and Costs.
- Recommendations.
- Validation.
- Sponsors.

A summary of the information in each section follows, along with the abstract of the guideline on breastfeeding that we used as our clinical example at the start of the chapter.[4]

Objective

The purpose of this section is to provide key information for the readers to decide if the guideline is relevant. The *Objective* identifies the health problem (disease or condition) that the guideline includes; the health care strategies that will address the problem; the patients to whom the guideline applies; and the care providers who are expected to use the guideline.

"To assess the benefits of breast feeding and to make recommendations for encouraging Canadian women to breast feed their infants. These recommendations specifically refer to care given during periodic health examinations (PHEs) in primary care settings and are for use by health professionals and health care planners."

Options

The purpose is to identify the key health care options so that the reader can determine whether the guideline is relevant. It identifies the health care options that will be examined in the guideline. Often these are just listed, and will be addressed later under the *Benefits, Harms, and Costs* section.

"Interventions to encourage breast feeding include breast feeding classes, individual teaching, nursing immediately after delivery (early contact), avoidance of bottle supplementation, and avoidance of provision of infant formula samples at birth."

Outcomes

The purpose is to identify the main outcomes considered in the guideline. The *Outcomes* section includes health outcomes, often in order of importance (mortality, morbidity, signs and symptoms, health care use, health-related behaviors, and quality of life), along with the main economic outcomes, and outcomes related to health care procedures or tests.

"Gastrointestinal and respiratory infections, otitis media, atopic disease, diabetes mellitus, infant body weight, maternal bonding, and duration of breast feeding."

Evidence

The purpose of this section is to provide information on the guideline development process so that a reader can decide if he or she is confident that the collection and synthesis methods included key relevant studies. The *Evidence* section includes methods for collecting the evidence (search methods), search results, methods for combining and analyzing the evidence, methods for assessing the strength of evidence, and planned updates or reviews.

"MEDLINE was searched up to December 1993 with the terms breast feeding, counselling, infections, allergy, nutrition, and infant development. Bibliographies of relevant papers were also checked. Studies with clinical outcomes that evaluated mothers and children in developed countries were selected. Study results were synthesized in table or graphic format only. Quality of evidence was rated according to 5 levels and recommendations were graded into 5 categories."

Values

This section provides an idea of the perspective taken during guideline development, and includes a list of major organizations involved, panel membership, methods or synthesizing panel member opinions or disagreements, and panel point of view and preferences.

"The 13-member Task Force of experts in family medicine, geriatric medicine, pediatrics, psychiatry and epidemiology used an evidence-based method for evaluating the effectiveness of preventive health care interventions. Recommendations were not based on cost-effectiveness of options. Patient preferences were not discussed.

Background papers providing critical appraisal of the evidence and tentative recommendations prepared by the chapter author were pre-circulated to the members. Evidence for this topic was presented and deliberated upon in 1- to 2-day meetings, 2 to 3 times per year from June 1993 to January 1994.

Consensus was reached on final recommendations."

Benefits, Harms, and Costs

This section presents evidence on the effect of the various options on the specified outcomes. It includes potential benefits of options and the magnitude for the benefits, potential harms of the options, and the magnitude of the harms, and any cost analyses. It is often one of the longest sections of the abstract or original guideline.

"1 systematic review from 1986 found no differences in infections in participants in developed countries for any outcomes measured for breast fed infants. Since then 1 British cohort study found fewer gastrointestinal and respiratory infections. 1 Danish study found no differences, and a third cohort study found that infants who were exclusively breast fed for 4 or more months were protected against acute (odds ratio [OR] 0.72) and recurrent otitis media (OR 0.54).

Several cohort studies and 1 RCT found no increase in length of time to development of atopy in preterm infants although 1 study found infants who were at risk for atopy (positive family history or positive cord blood for immunoglobulin E) were protected with breast feeding. Dietary restrictions for the mother may also protect against atopy in infants who are breast fed (1 cohort and 2 trials).

Case-control studies have shown breast feeding protects against the development of diabetes mellitus, particularly in persons who have genetic markers for the development of diabetes. Growth and development are not affected by breast feeding although some studies show lower body weight and higher intelligence in infants who were breast fed. Studies of maternal bonding have inconclusive data on the importance of breast feeding. 1 meta-analysis (2 RCTs) of breast feeding education showed higher rates of breast feeding with education. An RCT found individual teaching was more effective than group teaching for increasing the rates of breast feeding. Postnatal support reduced the OR to 0.75 (95% CI 0.62 to 0.91) for stopping breast feeding. 1 RCT of early contact found breast feeding to be a median of 77 days longer when early contact occurred. A small Canadian study found early contact increased the rate of breast feeding continuation (60% vs 20%, P < 0.001) at the end of the study. 2 other studies had mixed results although a meta-analysis showed an overall increase in breast feeding with early contact. Bottle supplementation studies were difficult to interpret. 2 RCTs found free samples distributed during hospital stay decreased the rate of breast feeding at 2 or 3 months."

Recommendations

This section presents the recommendations made by the guideline developers. It lists recommendations with assigned grades, evidence levels, or both. A "good" guideline will include supporting citations linked to individual recommendations.

"Level of evidence [I, II-1, II-2, II-3, III] and grade [A, B, C, D, E] are indicated after each recommendation. Citations supporting individual recommendations are identified in the guideline text.

1. *There is good evidence to counsel women to breast feed their infants [II-2, A].*
2. *There is good evidence to implement peripartum interventions (early, frequent mother-infant contact; rooming in; and banning provision of free formula samples) that promote breast feeding [I, A]."*

Validation

This section provides information on the involvement of outside agencies and people, what contribution they made to its development with respect to their values, and their refinement of the guideline and its developmental process. It includes a description of external peer review before publication, external pilot testing before publication, and agreement and disagreement of recommendations with those in other guidelines.

"Recommendations and background papers were sent for external peer review. The American Academy of Pediatrics and the Canadian Pediatrics Society recommended breast feeding as the preferred method of infant feeding plus encouraged public education programs, promotion of breast feeding at prenatal visits and during maternity ward care, and provision of facilities to allow breast feeding at work and day care centres. The World Health Organization and the UNICEF encourage breast feeding and support the above mentioned programs."

Sponsors

The purpose of this section is to identify the sponsoring and endorsing agencies and thus provide information on potential biases and special interests the guideline developers might have had.

"The Canadian Task Force on the Periodic Health Examination developed this guideline with funding from Health Canada."

Summary

Guidelines are additions important to the health care literature and for patient care-decision making. They engender feelings of support and condemnation, but are probably here to stay. The Evidence-Based Medicine Working Group in their Users' Guides[16] suggests that the following aspects of guidelines are important: the inclusion of clearly specified, important options and outcomes; an explicit and sensible process used to identify, select and combine evidence; explicit and sensible processes used to assess the relative value of different outcomes; accounting for important recent developments; and subjection to peer review and testing.

RETRIEVAL

Citations of guidelines published in medical journals are searchable in MEDLINE and other general-purpose and specialty databases. They have recently become easier to search in MEDLINE and its related databases, such as HealthStar, with the use of the publication types GUIDELINE for administrative or procedural guidelines, and PRACTICE GUIDELINE for specific health care guidelines. Furthermore, the National Library of Medicine database HealthSTAR contains practice guidelines, and health services, quality improvement and assessment literature from MEDLINE, and health technology assessment articles not indexed in other MEDLINE databases. CINAHL is a rich database for this material, and includes the full text of many clinical practice guidelines. The Internet also has many good listings of clinical practice guidelines. One excellent one is published by the Canadian Medical Association at *http://www.cma.ca/cpgs/index.htm*. They have a listing of more than 500 clinical practice guidelines, and have made a strong comitment to keeping the listing up-to-date. The AHCPR in conjunction with the American Medical Association and the American Association of Health Plans also has a strong listing of clinical practice guidelines at *http://www.guidelines.gov/*.

MEDLINE

MeSH, Subheading, Publication Types, and Textwords for Clinical Practice Guidelines

MeSH
Guidelines
    Practice guidelines
Consensus development conferences
    Consensus development conferences, NIH

Publication Types
Guideline (pt)
    Practice guideline (pt)
Consensus development conference (pt)
    Consensus development conference, NIH (pt)

Subheadings
Standards

Textwords
Guideline:
Recommend:
Consensus
Standard:
Parameter
Position paper

Please feel free to use some or all of the other names listed earlier in this chapter.

CINAHL Database for Nursing and Allied Health Literature

CINAHL Index Terms and Document Types for Clinical Practice Guidelines

CINAHL Index Terms
Practice guidelines

CINAHL Subheadings
Standards

CINAHL Document types
Practice guidelines
Nursing interventions

Textwords
Use list from MEDLINE

All extracts from the CINAHL® Thesaurus Copyright © 1999, Cinahl Information Systems. Reprinted with permission from Cinahl Information Systems.

PsycINFO

Index Terms for Clinical Practice Guidelines

Index Terms
Professional standards
Professional ethics
Quality of services

Textwords
Use list from MEDLINE

EMBASE/EXCERPTA MEDICA

Index Terms, Links, and EMTAGS for Clinical Practice Guidelines

Index Terms
Practice guideline
    Clinical pathway
    Clinical protocol
    Good clinical practice
Treatment outcome
    Outcomes research
    Treatment failure

Textwords
Use list from MEDLINE

EXAMPLES

Example 7–1
Solomon MJ, McLeod RS. Periodic health examination, 1994 update: 2. Screening strategies for colorectal cancer. Canadian Task Force on the Periodic Health Examination. CMAJ 1994;152:154–8.

This guideline was produced for the Canadian Task Force on the Periodic Health Examination and published in CMAJ. Note MEDLINE search with terms *screening* and *colorectal neoplasia*. Indexing is poor, probably because it is an older guideline. The clinical bottom line seems to be that unless you have risk factors such as family history, you probably do not need to be screened for colorectal cancer.

Retrieval Can Be Done Using Any of the Following:

MeSH indexing	—no indexing for retrieval
Textwords	Periodic health examination (title and abstract)
	Recommendations (abstract)
	Canadian Task Force (title and abstract)

Example 7–2
Kesaniemi YA. Guidelines for methods to determine efficacy and safety of drugs acting on the gastrointestinal tract. The International Union of Pharmacology (IUPHAR). Am J Cardiol 1998;81(8A):27F–8F.

This is not an evidence-based recommendation, nor one produced by an organization or group of experts, although Dr. Kesaniemi is considered an expert in his field. The author makes broad statements and recommendations backed up with almost no evidence. No methods section for how the guideline was formed, or on what the recommendations are based, is included, and the bibliography is short.

Retrieval Can Be Done Using Any of the Following:

MeSH indexing	guideline (publication type)
Textwords	guidelines (title) **note no abstract

MEDLINE Record for Example 7–1

Unique Identifier   94258632

Authors   Solomon MJ. McLeod RS.

Institution   Department of Surgery, University of Toronto, Ont.

Title   Periodic health examination, 1994 update: 2. Screening strategies for colorectal cancer. Canadian Task Force on the Periodic Health Examination [see comments].

Source   CMAJ. 150(12):1961–70, 1994 Jun 15.

MeSH Subject Headings

Adult
Aged
Aged, 80 and over
Canada/ep [Epidemiology]

Colonoscopy
Colorectal Neoplasms/di [Diagnosis]
Colorectal Neoplasms/ep [Epidemiology]
*Colorectal Neoplasms/pc [Prevention & Control]
Human
Incidence

*Mass Screening/mt [Methods]
Middle Age
Occult Blood
*Physical Examination/mt
    [Methods]
Predictive Value of Tests
Public Health
Risk Factors
Sensitivity and Specificity
Sigmoidoscopy
Support, Non-U.S. Gov't

Abstract
OBJECTIVE: To make recommendations on the effectiveness of screening for colorectal cancer in asymptomatic patients over 40 years of age. OPTIONS: Multiphase screening that begins with test for fecal occult blood, uniphase screening with sigmoidoscopy and uniphase screening with colonoscopy. Options included screening repeated at different intervals and different procedures for patients with selected risk factors. OUTCOMES: Rates of death, death from cancer and cancer detection; compliance, feasibility and accuracy of each manoeuvre. EVIDENCE: A MEDLINE search for articles published between January 1966 and June 1993 with the use of MeSH terms "screening" and "colorectal neoplasia," a check with the reference sections of review articles published before June 1993 and a survey of content experts. Articles were weighted according to the Canadian Task Force on the Periodic Health Examination levels of evidence. VALUES: The highest value was assigned to manoeuvres that lowered the rate of death from cancer and had a low rate of false-positive results and acceptable cost and compliance. Recommendations were determined by consensus of the authors, members of the task force and colorectal cancer experts. BENEFITS, HARMS AND COSTS: There is evidence that annual fecal occult blood testing with the use of the rehydrated Hemoccult test has a small but significant benefit in lowering the rate of death from cancer after more than 10 years of screening; however, the high rate of false-positive results (9.8%) and the poor sensitivity of annual (49%) and biennial (38%) screening make this a poor method for detecting colorectal cancer. There is fair evidence that screening with sigmoidoscopy may improve survival rates; however, this may be due to volunteer bias. The high cost of and poor compliance with colonoscopic screening make this an unfeasible strategy.

Publication Type   Journal Article

MEDLINE Record for Example 7–2

Unique Identifier   98265937

Authors   Kesaniemi YA.

Institution   Department of Internal Medicine and Biocenter Oulu, University of Oulu, Finland.

Title   Guidelines for methods to determine efficacy and safety of drugs acting on the gastrointestinal tract. The international union of pharmacology (IUPHAR). [Review] [6 refs]

Source   American Journal of Cardiology. 81(8A):27F–28F, 1998 Apr 23.

MeSH Subject Headings
Antilipemic Agents/ae [Adverse Effects]
*Antilipemic Agents/pd [Pharmacology]
Cardiovascular Diseases/pc [Prevention & Control]
Diet
*Drug Evaluation/mt [Methods]
Drugs, Investigational/ae [Adverse Effects]
*Drugs, Investigational/pd [Pharmacology]
Female
*Gastrointestinal System/de [Drug Effects]
Gastrointestinal System/me [Metabolism]
Human
Hyperlipidemia/dt [Drug Therapy]
Intestinal Absorption/de [Drug Effects]
Lipids/me [Metabolism]
Male
Patient Selection
Safety

Publication Type   Guideline. Journal Article. Review. Review, Tutorial.

Example 7–3
Moutquin JM, Garner PR, Burrows RF, et al. Report of the Canadian Hypertension Society Consensus Conference: 2. Nonpharmacologic management and prevention of hypertensive disorders in pregnancy. CMAJ 1997;157:907–19.

This is a new guideline, and the textwords and indexing are exemplary. The guideline is an important one because of the clinical importance to the mother and child of gestational hypertension. It is also strongly evidence-based.

Retrieval Can Be Done Using Any of the Following:

MeSH indexing	Consensus development conference (publication type)
	Guideline (publication type)
	Practice guideline (publication type)
Textwords	Consensus conference (title)
	Guidelines (abstract)
	Cochrane database of systematic reviews (abstract)
	MEDLINE (abstract)
	Randomized trials (abstract)
	Consensus (abstract)
	All structured abstract headings

Example 7–4
Guidelines for counseling postmenopausal women about preventive hormone therapy. American College of Physicians. Ann Intern Med. 1992;117:1038-41.
Grady D, Rubin SM, Petitti DB, et al Hormone therapy to prevent disease and prolong life in postmenopausal women. Ann Intern Med 1992;117:1016–37.

This pair of articles from the same issue of *Annals of Internal Medicine* provides the evidence and the guideline itself for use by clinicians and patients. Indexing for the systematic review is usual. Note that the numbering in the guideline does not refer to recommendation strength or grading, but to sections in the systematic review. Data from these two publications have been heavily used in many decisions on whether to take hormone replacement therapy during and after menopause.

Retrieval Can Be Done Using Any of the Following:

MeSH indexing	Guideline (publication type)
	Practice guideline (publication type)
Textwords	Guidelines (title)
	—note no abstract

MEDLINE Record for Example 7–3

Unique Identifier 97468735

Authors Moutquin JM. Garner PR. Burrows RF. Rey E. Helewa ME. Lange IR. Rabkin SW.

Institution Department of Obstetrics and Gynecology, Laval University, Sainte-Foy, Que.

Title Report of the Canadian Hypertension Society **Consensus Conference**: 2. Nonpharmacologic management and prevention of hypertensive disorders in pregnancy. [Review] [105 refs]

Source CMAJ. 157(7):907–19, 1997 Oct 1.

MeSH Subject Headings
Female
Human
*Hypertension/th [Therapy]
Pregnancy

*Pregnancy Complications,
  Cardiovascular/th [Therapy]
Support, Non-U.S. Gov't

Abstract
OBJECTIVE: To provide Canadian physicians with comprehensive, evidence-based **guidelines** for the nonpharmacologic management and prevention of gestational hypertension and pre-existing hypertension during pregnancy. OPTIONS: Lifestyle modifications, dietary or nutrient interventions, plasma volume expansion and use of prostaglandin precursors or inhibitors. OUTCOMES: In gestational hypertension, prevention of complications and death related to either its occurrence (primary or secondary prevention) or its severity (tertiary prevention). In pre-existing hypertension, prevention of superimposed gestational hypertension and intrauterine growth retardation. EVIDENCE: Articles retrieved from the pregnancy and childbirth module of the **Cochrane Database of Systematic Reviews**; pertinent articles published from 1966 to 1996, retrieved through **a** MEDLINE search; and review of original randomized trials from 1942 to 1996. If evidence was unavailable, consensus was reached by the members of the consensus panel set up by the Canadian Hypertension Society. VALUES: High priority was given to prevention of adverse maternal and neonatal outcomes in pregnancies with established hypertension and in those at high risk of gestational hypertension through the provision of effective nonpharmacologic management. BENEFITS, HARMS AND COSTS: Reduction in rate of long-term hospital admissions among women with gestational hypertension, with establishment of safe home-care blood pressure monitoring and appropriate rest. Targeting prophylactic interventions in selected high-risk groups may avoid ineffective use in the general population. Cost was not considered. RECOMMENDATION: Nonpharmacologic management should be considered for pregnant women with a systolic blood pressure of 140-150 mm Hg or a diastolic pressure of 90-99 mm Hg, or both, measured in a clinical setting. A short-term hospital stay may be required for diagnosis and for ruling out severe gestational hypertension (preeclampsia). In the latter case, the only effective treatment is delivery. Palliative management, dependent on blood pressure, gestational age and presence of associated maternal and fetal risk factors, includes close supervision, limitation of activities and some bed rest. A normal diet without salt restriction is advised. Promising preventive interventions that may reduce the incidence of gestational hypertension, especially with proteinuria, include calcium supplementation (2 g/d), fish oil supplementation and low-dose acetylsalicylic acid therapy, particularly in women at high risk for early-onset gestational hypertension. Pre-existing hypertension should be managed the same way as before pregnancy. However, additional concerns are the effects on fetal well-being and the worsening of hypertension during the second half of pregnancy. There is, as yet, no treatment that will prevent exacerbation of the condition. VALIDATION: The guidelines share the principles in consensus reports from the US and Australia on the nonpharmacologic management of hypertension in pregnancy. [References: 105]

Publication Type **Consensus Development Conference. Guideline.** Journal Article. **Practice Guideline.** Review.

MEDLINE Record for Example 7–4a

Unique Identifier   93073344

Authors   Anonymous.

Title   Guidelines for counseling postmenopausal women about preventive hormone therapy. American College of Physicians [comment] [see comments].

Source   Annals of Internal Medicine. 117(12):1038–41, 1992 Dec 15.

MeSH Subject Headings
Counseling
Estrogen Replacement Therapy/ae [Adverse Effects]
*Estrogen Replacement Therapy
Female
Human
Middle Age
Progestational Hormones/ad [Administration & Dosage]
Risk Factors

Publication Type   Comment. **Guideline.** Journal Article. Practice Guideline.

MEDLINE Record for Example 7–4b

Unique Identifier   93073343

Authors   Grady D. Rubin SM. Petitti DB. Fox CS. Black D. Ettinger B. Ernster VL. Cummings SR.

Institution   University of California, Prevention Sciences Group, San Francisco 94105.

Title   Hormone therapy to prevent disease and prolong life in postmenopausal women [see comments]. [Review] [265 refs]

Source   Annals of Internal Medicine. 117(12):1016–37, 1992 Dec 15.

MeSH Subject Headings
Breast Neoplasms/ep [Epidemiology]
Cerebrovascular Disorders/ep [Epidemiology]
Coronary Disease/ep [Epidemiology]
Endometrial Neoplasms/ci [Chemically Induced]
Estrogen Replacement Therapy/ae [Adverse Effects]
*Estrogen Replacement Therapy
Female
Hip Fractures/pc [Prevention & Control]
Human
Middle Age
Progestational Hormones/ad [Administration & Dosage]
Risk Factors
Support, Non-U.S. Gov't

Abstract
PURPOSE: To critically review the risks and benefits of hormone therapy for asymptomatic postmenopausal women who are considering long-term hormone therapy to prevent disease or to prolong life. DATA SOURCES: Review of the English-language literature since 1970 on the effect of estrogen therapy and estrogen plus progestin therapy on endometrial cancer, breast cancer, coronary heart disease, osteoporosis, and stroke. We used standard meta-analytic statistical methods to pool estimates from studies to determine summary relative risks for these diseases in hormone users and modified lifetable methods to estimate changes in lifetime probability and life expectancy due to use of hormone regimens. RESULTS: There is evidence that estrogen therapy decreases risk for coronary heart disease and for hip fracture, but long-term estrogen therapy increases risk for endometrial cancer and may be associated with a small increase in risk for breast cancer. The increase in endometrial cancer risk can probably be avoided by adding a progestin to the estrogen regimen for women who have a uterus, but the effects of combination hormones on risk for other diseases has not been adequately studied. We present estimates for changes in lifetime probabilities of disease and life expectancy due to hormone therapy in women who have had a hysterectomy; with coronary heart disease; and at increased risk for coronary heart disease, hip fracture, and breast cancer. CONCLUSIONS: Hormone therapy should probably be recommended for women who have had a hysterectomy and for those with coronary heart disease or at high risk for coronary heart disease. For other women, the best course of action is unclear. [References: 265]

Publication Type   Journal Article. Review. Review, Academic.

ASSIGNMENT

Try the MEDLINE and HealthStar databases, and any other source you can think of.

1. Many national and international guidelines exist for cholesterol testing and treatments. How many can you find?

REFERENCES

1. Field MJ, Lohr KN. Clinical practice guidelines. Washington, DC: National Academy Press; 1990.
2. American Medical Association. Directory of practice parameters: titles, sources and updates. Chicago: American Medical Association; 1996.
3. ECRI. Health Care Standards, 1997. Plymouth Meeting, PA: ECRI; 1997.
4. Wang EL. Breast feeding. In: Canadian Task Force on the Periodic Health Examination. Canadian Guide to Clinical Preventive Health Care. Ottawa: Health Canada; 1994. p. 232–42.
5. Hayward RS, Guyatt GH, Moore KA, et al. Canadian physicians' attitudes about and preferences regarding clinical practice guidelines. CMAJ 1997;156:1715–23.
6. Canadian Task Force on the Periodic Health Examination. Canadian Guide to Clinical Preventive Health Care. Ottawa: Health Canada; 1994.
7. U.S. Preventive Services Task Force. Guide to Clinical Preventive Services. 2nd ed. Baltimore: Williams & Wilkins; 1996.
8. Atkins S, Karmerow D, Eisenberg JM. Evidence-based medicine at the Agency for Health Care Policy and Research. ACP J Club 1998 Mar–Apr:128:A14–6.
9. Woolf SH. Can clinical practice guidelines define good medical care? The need for good science and the disclosure of uncertainty when defining "best practices." Chest 1998;13:1663–71S.
10. Heffner JE. Does evidence-based medicine help the development of clinical practice guidelines? Chest 1998;113:172S–8S.
11. Carruthers SG, Larochelle P, Haynes RB, et al. Report of the Canadian Hypertension Concensus Conference: 1 Introduction. CMAJ 1993;149:289–93.
12. Solomon MJ, McLeod RS. Periodic health examination, 1994 update: 2. Screening strategies for colorectal cancer. Canadian Task Force on the Periodic Health Examination. CMAJ 1994;152:154–8.
13. Audet A, Greenfield S, Field M. Medical practice guidelines: current activities and future directions. Ann Intern Med 1990;113:709–14.
14. B.C. Office of Health Technology Assessment Centre for Health Services and Policy Research. Bone mineral density testing: does the evidence support its selective use in well women? Vancouver, British Columbia; University of British Columbia; 1997. p. 130–1.
15. Hayward RSW, Wilson MC, Tunis SR, et al. More informative abstracts of articles describing clinical practice guidelines. Ann Intern Med 1993;118:731–7.
16. Richardson WS, Detsky AS for the Evidence-Based Medicine Working Group. Users' guides to the medical literature. VII. How to use a clinical decision analysis. A. Are the results of the study valid? JAMA 1995;273:1292–5.

8

Secondary Publications: Economic Analyses

Angela Eady, BA, MLS

That resources in health care are unavoidably finite has highlighted the importance of decisions about resource allocation. Health care professionals may participate in such decisions, which means they have to consider not only the effectiveness but also the costs of the screening (mammograms for breast cancer), diagnostic (magnetic resonance imaging for multiple sclerosis), therapeutic (defibrillators for coronary heart disease), and preventive (assertiveness training programs to prevent teen pregnancy) interventions they choose. One tool that helps delineate the benefits and costs of a health care procedure or treatment is an **economic analysis**, which uses formal quantitative methods to compare alternative interventions for their resource use and outcomes achieved. Ideally, economic analyses can help to identify wasteful, ineffective procedures and less-costly interventions that are as effective as high-cost ones.[1] The task is often more complex, however, because more effective interventions may be more costly, and certain tradeoffs have to be considered. Not surprisingly, the number of economic analyses in the health care literature has grown in recent years.[2]

Various types of economic analyses are used; high-quality ones have some common elements. First, they compare alternative strategies of screening, treatment, prevention, quality improvement, or diagnosis; doing nothing may be considered an alternative strategy. Second, they include data on costs and benefits, both of which are required for a full economic comparison. If only costs are included, the comparison is called a **cost analysis**, and it does not help in formulating decisions about whether the intervention is an effective use of resources. Third, good economic analyses inform readers of the additional (or incremental) costs and benefits of one intervention over another.

Although good economic analyses share certain elements, they may differ in many other ways: for example, design, methods, type of costs used, and the perspective taken when comparing costs and benefits. Some economic analysts have used a cube drawing to represent three dimensions of a health economic analysis: the types of analysis, costs and benefits, and the point of view from which an economic analysis is done.[3] The cube drawing shows that all of these aspects intersect and must be considered in relation to one another. These dimensions are discussed below. The design, or overall structure, of economic analyses will also be discussed.

The differences across economic analyses arise from the decisions that investigators make when doing one. When analyzing costs and benefits for an intervention in a particular population, investigators often make assumptions about costs or benefits, and these may vary across different situations. In good economic analyses, *sensitivity analyses* will be used to see whether these assumptions have an influence on the results. (See Chapter 6 Secondary Publications: Systematic Reviews for a discussion on sensitivity analyses.)

ECONOMIC ANALYSIS DESIGNS

Designs for economic analyses include: randomized controlled trials; systematic reviews of cost-effectiveness analyses; retrospective analyses of a published randomized controlled trial; and decision models that use data from trials or systematic reviews to estimate the outcomes for a hypothetical group of patients. When data from previously published trials are used in an economic analysis, the methodology of those studies will influence the validity of the economic analysis.

TYPES OF ECONOMIC ANALYSES

How interventions are compared in an analysis will depend on the way benefits and costs are measured and valued.[4] As has already been mentioned, a cost analysis, which may also be called a *cost minimization analysis*[4] or a *cost identification analysis*,[3] considers costs only. This type of analysis is fairly basic, and is only useful insofar as the intervention is known to be equivalent or superior to the comparison intervention. In these cases, a cost analysis can show whether an effective intervention is less costly than interventions used in standard care. For example, Covinsky et al. compared the costs of caring for medical patients on a special unit designed to help older people maintain or achieve independence in self-care activities with the costs of usual care.[5] They used a randomized controlled trial and reported the health outcomes as well. Patients in the special unit spent less time in the hospital and were less likely to need home nursing. The re-admission rates and caregiver strain scores were similar for both groups of patients. Given that the special unit was more effective for improving some outcomes and similar to standard care for all other outcomes, the costs can be compared. The authors found that the two interventions did not differ substantially in costs ($6608 total cost to care for patients in the special unit, compared with $7240 total cost to care for patients on the usual-care ward).

More often, though, new therapies, diagnostic tests, or health care procedures are more effective *and* more expensive. For analyzing the costs and benefits of these interventions (and for including data on benefits as well as costs), a finer level of analysis is required. Cost-benefit analyses, cost-effectiveness analyses, and cost-utility analyses are more sophisticated methods of comparing costs and benefits.

A **cost-benefit analysis** expresses all costs and benefits in monetary terms. The difference between the benefit (in monetary units) and the costs is called the *net benefit*. Interventions are considered favorable when their benefits exceed their costs (that is, a positive net benefit). For example, Golaszewski et al. did a cost-benefit analysis of a major health program in the workplace called the "Taking Care Program."[6] The Travelers Insurance Company introduced this program to its 36,000 employees and retirees in the U.S. The program consisted of a health risk appraisal, medical reference text, monthly health newsletter, several program introduction videotapes, and media blitzes (called "FOCUS programs") on selected health topics. Employees helped to implement the program. Golaszewski et al. calculated the costs of the program and translated the benefits into costs. They did this by estimating the costs of health care, absenteeism, death benefits that were paid out by the company, productivity gains, and income generated by the program through membership fees. They found that the Taking Care Program led to a net value—the total program effects minus costs—of $72.35 million, which translated into a benefit-cost ratio of 3:4.

Researchers often find it difficult to express outcomes in health care as monetary values. Cost-effectiveness and cost-utility analyses allow researchers to analyze benefits and costs without having to convert benefits into monetary values, and consequently these are more common in the health care literature.[2] The choice of a cost-effectiveness or cost-utility analysis will depend on the types of outcomes of interest.

If the interventions have the same health outcome, then a **cost-effectiveness analysis** can be done. It shows what the additional cost is for the additional improvement in health achieved by using one intervention rather than another. For example, Salzmann et al. wanted to determine whether it would be cost-effective to extend screening recommendations to include mammograms for women 40 to 49 years of age.[7] The outcome in this study was reduced mortality, which was measured for three screening strategies. The authors did a cost-effectiveness analysis to compare the cost per life saved for biennially screening women from 50 to 69 years of age compared with: 1) no screening; and 2) screening women every 18 months from 40 to 49 years of age, followed by screening biennially from 50 to 69 years age. They found that screening women 50 years and older cost $21,400 for each year of life saved, whereas extending screening to include women 40 to 49 years of age cost $105,000 for each year of life saved.

Interventions can affect patients' quality of life as well as their health outcomes. The different effects of an intervention make it difficult to do a cost-effectiveness analysis. In these instances, **cost-utility analyses** are used, which incorporate patient preferences for the types of interventions that are being compared. Cost-utility analyses report the number of years of life saved, which are adjusted for quality (these are also known as quality-adjusted life years [QALY] gained). Glennie interviewed seven patients with schizophrenia to collect data on patient preferences for the use of clozapine and risperidone compared with haloperidol.[8] She found that risperidone led to $6500 saved per year with a gain of 0.04 QALY, and clozapine led to $39,000 saved per year with a gain of 0.04 QALY.

Although economic analysts distinguish among the four different types of analysis, the terminology for economic analyses in the health care literature is not so neatly classified. The label of cost-benefit analysis is applied broadly. In a review of studies in MEDLINE, *Current Contents*, and HealthSTAR, Zarnke et al. found that 53% of the 95 studies that were labeled as cost-benefit analyses did not evaluate health outcomes.[9] Also, only 32% of the 95 studies were bona fide cost-benefit analyses: that is, health outcomes were translated into monetary values in them.

TYPES OF COSTS

Various costs are associated with the use of an intervention: some obvious and some less so. The types of costs included in an economic analysis will depend on the perspective taken, and this is discussed in the next section. Costs can be classified as direct or indirect. **Direct costs** include costs of providing medical care (for example, intervention costs and the health care professionals' salaries) and nonmedical costs to patients and families (for example, patients' cost of transportation to the medical facility, and other such costs associated with illness and the receipt of medical care). **Indirect costs** include the broader costs of illness (for example, time lost from work) or mortality (for example, premature death leading to removal of that person from the workforce).

Economic analyses describe the types of costs and how they are measured. Changes in the value of money over time are taken into consideration. For some interventions, like screening, the benefits occur in the future. To determine the present value of these future costs, discount rates are used. Generally, these discount rates range from 2 to 6%. Salzmann and colleagues report that they included three costs in their analysis of breast cancer screening strategies: the cost of screening mammographic examinations, the cost of evaluating abnormal mammograms, and the cost of treating breast cancer.[7] These direct costs were measured in U.S. dollars, which were inflated to 1995 dollars by using the consumer price index for medical services. The authors also discounted costs at a rate of 3% per year. Rosenheck et al. included nonmedical costs in their study on clozapine in patients with schizophrenia, which were the costs of the criminal justice system (police contacts and arrests) and the administrative costs of transfer payments (programs that provide welfare or disability payments to patients).[10] Indirect costs were also included: loss of productivity (loss of earnings from employment) and family burden (days lost by family members from work and from unpaid domestic activity because of caring for the patient). They found that clozapine was more effective than haloperidol for patients with schizophrenia, with similar costs for both drugs. However, as Jones pointed out in a commentary, costs to the community may grow as patients with schizophrenia get better and start using services that were not of benefit to them before.[11] An economic analysis that includes the costs of community services would need to be done to see whether societal costs are increased by the use of clozapine.

THE PERSPECTIVE OF AN ECONOMIC ANALYSIS

Economic analyses are always done from a particular viewpoint. The perspective can be that of the patient, the payer, the health care provider, or society. The cost-effectiveness of an intervention can change when analyzed from a different perspective. For example, when Anis et al. analyzed the cost-effectiveness of cyclosporine in patients with rheumatoid arthritis from the perspective of the Ontario Ministry of Health (payer), they found that the incremental cost of using cyclosporine rather than placebo was $11,547 per patient each year.[12] From a societal perspective, however, the incremental cost was greater: $20,698 per patient each year. Some of the costs included in the analysis from the societal perspective were over-the-counter medication costs, the cost of home-visiting nurse services, and time lost from work.

TESTING THE ASSUMPTIONS OF AN ECONOMIC ANALYSIS

Economic analysts often make assumptions. These assumptions may include costs, the methods used to measure an outcome, discount rates, and estimates of the intervention's effect. The assumptions inherent in an economic analysis may influence the results, and show that it is sensitive to certain factors. A **sensitivity analysis** will help determine whether the results of an economic analysis are consistent or whether they require certain assumptions to be true. Sometimes economic analysts will use the 95% confidence intervals associated with the effects of an intervention to determine whether the results remain the same across different estimates of the effect.

In an economic analysis by Lave et al., three different depression treatments were compared: psychotherapy, drug treatment (nortriptyline), and usual care by a primary care physician.[13] The authors calculated the cost for each additional depression-free day experienced by patients using the results from one of two scales to measure depression. They found that psychotherapy and nortriptyline were both more effective and more expensive than usual care. However, when they used the results from the second depression scale in the analysis, the effect was no longer statistically significant for psychotherapy. The analysis was sensitive to the type of scale used to measure depression.

SUMMARY

Economic analyses analyze the costs in relation to the benefits of an intervention. Data on benefits *and* costs are important for evaluating whether an intervention is an effective and efficient use of resources. Economic analyses should compare alternative strategies for diagnosis, therapy, prevention, or quality improvement, and they should also provide information about the additional, or incremental, costs and benefits of using one strategy (or intervention) over another. The methods used to evaluate the benefits of an intervention will influence its validity, which means that the trials or reviews used to obtain data should meet the criteria for therapy, diagnosis, or quality improvement trials, depending on which intervention is being studied. Different types of costs—direct and indirect—are used in economic analyses. The different methods of analyzing costs in relation to benefits are cost-analyses (costs only are considered, so this type of analysis is useful only when the effectiveness of an intervention is known to be equivalent or superior to the alternative); cost-benefit analyses (the costs and benefits of an intervention are measured by using monetary values); cost-effectiveness analyses (the cost of the additional health improvement is calculated); and cost-utility analyses (the patient's quality of life is incorporated into the analysis, and the cost for each QALY is calculated). The health care literature does not differentiate clearly between cost analyses, cost-benefit analyses, and cost-effectiveness analyses. Economic analysts make assumptions about many aspects of an analysis, including costs and benefits; and when uncertainty exists in an economic analysis, sensitivity analyses are used to determine whether the results depend on certain assumptions being true.

MEDLINE

MeSH, Subheadings, and Textwords for Economic Analyses

MeSH
Costs and cost analysis
    Cost allocation
    Cost-benefit analysis
    Cost control
        Cost savings
    Cost of illness
    Cost sharing
        Deductibles and coinsurance
    Health care costs
        Direct service costs
        Drug costs
        Employer health costs
        Hospital costs
    Health expenditures
        Capital expenditures

Subheading
Economics

Textwords
Cost:
Economic

CINAHL Database of Nursing and Allied Health Literature

CINAHL Index Terms and Subheadings for Economic Analyses

CINAHL Index terms
Costs and cost analysis
    Case mix
    Cost benefit analysis
    Cost Control
        Cost savings
    Diagnosis-related groups
    Health care costs
        Hospital costs
        Nursing costs

Resource allocation
    Health resource allocation

CINAHL Subheading
Economics

Textwords
Use MEDLINE selected above

CINAHL thesaurus terms provided by Katy Nesbit
All extracts from the CINAHL® Thesaurus Copyright © 1999, Cinahl Information Systems. Reprinted with permission from Cinahl Information Systems.

PsycINFO

Index Terms for Economic Analyses

Index terms
Cost and cost analyses
    Budgets
    Health care costs
Cost containment
Economics

Text words
Use same list as for MEDLINE

EMBASE/EXCERPTA MEDICA

Index Terms, Links, and EMTAGS for Economic Analyses

Index terms
Health economics
    Economic evaluation
        Cost benefit analysis
        Cost control
        Cost effectiveness analysis
        Cost minimization analysis
        Cost of illness
        Cost utility analysis
    Health care cost
      Drug cost
      Health care finacing
      Hospital cost
        Hospital finance
        Hospital purchasing
        Hospital running cost
Pharmacoeconomics
    Drug approval
    Drug cost
    Drug formulary
    Drug utilization
    Utilization review

Links (subheadings)
Pharmacoeconomics
Disease management

Emtags (publication types)
Economic aspect

MEDLINE HEDGES

No MEDLINE hedges have been developed yet for economic analyses.

EXAMPLES

Example 8–1
Randomized, controlled trial
Kraft MK, Rothbard AB, Hadley TR, et al. Are supplementary services provided during methadone maintenance really cost-effective? Am J Psychiatry 1997;154:1214–9.

This cost-effectiveness analysis uses data from a 24-week randomized, controlled trial. One hundred patients received methadone and were allocated to one of three support levels: minimum (methadone and one monthly counseling session); counseling (methadone and three counseling sessions each week plus behavioral interventions); or enhanced (methadone and seven counseling sessions each week plus extended onsite medical, psychiatric, employment, and family therapy services). Costs were measured by using the salary and benefits figures of the professional staff, average contact time for each treatment episode, and number and type of service contacts for each client. Kraft et al. found that the triweekly counseling sessions and behavioral interventions in addition to methadone were most cost-effective for abstinence from heroin and cocaine. The annual cost per abstinent client was $16,485 for minimum services, $9084 for counseling-and-methadone services, and $11,818 for enhanced services.

Retrieval Can Be Done Using Any of the Following:

MeSH indexing	Cost-benefit analysis
	Follow-up studies
	Health care costs
	Health services research
	Economics (subheading)
Textwords	Cost (title and abstract)
	Cost effectiveness (abstract)
	Cost effective (title)

Example 8–2
Systematic review
Stucki G, Johannesson M, Liang MG. Is misoprostol cost-effective in the prevention of nonsteroidal anti-inflammatory drug-induced gastropathy in patients with chronic arthritis? A review of conflicting economic evaluations. Arch Intern Med 1994;154:2020–5.

This review studied the cost-effectiveness of using misoprostol to prevent gastric problems in patients who used nonsteroidal anti-inflammatory drugs to control their arthritis. Five economic studies were identified. Each study used a different method for estimating the use of resources. Four studies found that misoprostol led to cost-savings and one study found that the costs were high for each life-year gained ($95,600) and each gas-

MEDLINE Record for Example 8–1

Unique Identifier   97432280

Authors   Kraft MK. Rothbard AB. Hadley TR. McLellan AT. Asch DA.

Institution   Rutgers University School of Social Work, Philadelphia, USA.

Title   Are supplementary services provided during methadone maintenance really cost-effective? [see comments].

Source   American Journal of Psychiatry. 154(9):1214–9, 1997 Sep.

MeSH Subject Headings

Adult	Human
Combined Modality Therapy	Male
Cost-Benefit Analysis	*Methadone/tu [Therapeutic Use]
*Counseling/ec [**Economics**]	Opioid-Related Disorders/ec [Economics]
Counseling/mt [Methods]	*Opioid-Related Disorders/rh [Rehabilitation]
Female	Support, Non-U.S. Gov't
Follow-Up Studies	Support, U.S. Gov't, Non-P.H.S.
Health Care Costs	Treatment Outcome
*Health Services Research	

Abstract

OBJECTIVE: Previous research has suggested that support services supplementing methadone maintenance programs vary in **their cost-effectiveness.** This study examined the cost-effectiveness of varying levels of supplementary support services to determine whether the relative cost-effectiveness of alternative levels of support is sustained over time. METHOD: A group of 100 methadone-maintained opiate users were randomly assigned to three treatment groups receiving different levels of support services during a 24-week clinical trial. One group received methadone treatment with a minimum of counseling, the second received methadone plus more intensive counseling, and the third received methadone plus enhanced counseling, medical, and psychosocial services. The results at the end of the trial period have been published elsewhere. This article reports the results of an analysis at a 6-month follow-up. RESULTS: The follow-up analysis reaffirmed the preliminary findings that the methadone plus counseling level provided the most cost-effective implementation of the treatment program. At 12 months, the annual cost per abstinent client was $16,485, $9,804, and $11,818 for the low, intermediate, and high levels of support, respectively. Abstinence rates were highest, but modestly so, for the group receiving the high-intensity, high-cost methadone with enhanced services intervention. CONCLUSIONS: This study suggests that large amounts of support to methadone-maintained clients are not cost-effective, but it also demonstrates that moderate amounts of support are better than minimal amounts. As funding for these programs is reduced, these findings suggest a floor below which supplementary support should not fall.

Publication Type   Journal Article.

MEDLINE Record for Example 8–2

Unique Identifier   94379874

Authors   Stucki G. Johannesson M. Liang MH.

Institution   Department of Health Policy and Management, Harvard School of Public Health, Boston, Massachusetts.

Title   Is misoprostol cost-effective in the prevention of nonsteroidal anti-inflammatory drug-induced gastropathy in patients with chronic arthritis? A review of conflicting economic evaluations [see comments]. [Review] [28 refs]

Source   Archives of Internal Medicine. 154(18):2020–5, 1994 Sep 26.

MeSH Subject Headings
*Anti-Inflammatory Agents, Non-Steroidal/ae [Adverse Effects]
Anti-Inflammatory Agents, Non-Steroidal/tu [Therapeutic Use]
*Arthritis/dt [Drug Therapy]
Cost-Benefit Analysis
Gastritis/ci [Chemically Induced]
*Gastritis/pc [Prevention & Control]
Human
*Misoprostol/ec [**Economics**]
Misoprostol/tu [Therapeutic Use]
Support, Non-U.S. Gov't
Support, U.S. Gov't, P.H.S.

Abstract
Whether misoprostol, a synthetic prostaglandin E1 analogue, should be routinely prescribed along with nonsteroidal anti-inflammatory drugs (NSAIDS) to prevent gastric damage is of great clinical importance and has profound cost implications. No consensus exists on whether misoprostol cotherapy results in a **cost-saving**, is **cost-effective**, or is costly. The different conclusions reached by five **economic** evaluations of misoprostol can be explained solely by the assumed absolute risk reduction of symptomatic ulcer, which was more than seven times greater in the studies that concluded that misoprostol was cost-effective than in a study that concluded misoprostol to be costly. Since no study has directly shown the effectiveness of misoprostol cotherapy in preventing clinically significant ulcer disease (ie, hemorrhage and perforation), it is impossible to judge which assumptions are most appropriate. The absence of firm data on the rate of NSAID-induced gastric ulcers reduced by misoprostol makes it impossible to conclude whether it is cost-effective in patients with chronic arthritis who use NSAIDS. [References: 28]

Publication Type   Journal Article. **Review.** Review, Tutorial.

---

tric bleed avoided ($5300). The results in each study that found misoprostol to be cost-saving were sensitive to a number of assumptions, including the cost of misoprostol, the number of patients who complied with treatment requirements, and the cost of ambulatory treatment. The conclusion of the study was that the diverse methods and conflicting results of the five economic evaluations reviewed do not provide a definitive answer to the question of whether misoprostol is cost-effective in patients with chronic arthritis.

Retrieval Can Be Done Using Any of the Following:

MeSH indexing	Cost-benefit analysis
	Economics (subheading)
	Review (publication type)
Textwords	Cost-effective (title and abstract)
	Cost-saving (abstract)
	Economic (title and abstract)

Example 8–3
Decision model
O'Brien B, Goeree R, Mohamed AH, Hunt R. Cost-effectiveness of *Helicobacter pylori* eradication for the long-term management of duodenal ulcer in Canada. Arch Intern Med 1995;155:1958–64.

O'Brien et al. used a decision-analysis model to determine the cost-effectiveness of eradicating a bacterium that is associated with the development of ulcers, *Helicobacter pylori (H. pylori)*. The authors compared three strategies: healing by immediately eradicating *H. pylori* with drugs; using ranitidine for healing and then eradicating *H. pylori* at recurrence; or using ranitidine for healing, maintenance therapy, and recurrences. They used a hypothetical cohort of patients whom they assumed had uncomplicated duodenal ulcers that had been confirmed by endoscopy. The authors used data from meta-analyses of randomized, controlled trials that studied alternative pharmacologic strategies for treating duodenal ulcers to calculate rates of recurrence. They calculated the costs of implementing each strategy for 12 months in the hypothetical cohort of patients. They found that immediate eradication of *H. pylori* was more cost-effective than eradication at recurrence or maintenance therapy with ranitidine. Sensitivity analyses did not change the ranking of alternatives.

Retrieval Can Be Done Using Any of the Following:

MeSH indexing	Cost-benefit analysis
	Decision support techniques
	Economics (subheading)
	Models, statistical

MEDLINE Record for Example 8–3

Unique Identifier 96006134

Authors O'Brien B. Goeree R. Mohamed AH. Hunt R.

Institution Department of Clinical Epidemiology and Biostatistics, McMaster University, Hamilton, Ontario.

Title **Cost-effectiveness** of *Helicobacter pylori* eradication for the long-term management of duodenal ulcer in Canada [see comments].

Source Archives of Internal Medicine. 155(18):1958–64, 1995 Oct 9.

MeSH Subject Headings

Canada	*Helicobacter Infections/ec [Economics]
Cost-Benefit Analysis	*Helicobacter Infections/th [Therapy]
*Decision Support Techniques	Human
*Duodenal Ulcer/ec [**Economics**]	**Models, Statistical**
Duodenal Ulcer/mi [Microbiology]	Recurrence
*Duodenal Ulcer/th [Therapy]	Support, Non-U.S. Gov't
*Helicobacter pylori	Time Factors

Abstract
BACKGROUND: A 1994 National Institutes of Health consensus panel recommended that eradication of *Helicobacter pylori* should be first-line therapy for persons with duodenal ulcer. OBJECTIVE: To assess the **cost-effectiveness** of *H pylori* eradication relative to alternative pharmacologic strategies in the long-term management of persons with confirmed duodenal ulcer. METHODS: **Decision analysis** model to estimate expected costs and symptomatic ulcer recurrences during a 12-month period for three general treatment strategies: (1) immediate *H pylori* eradication; (2) *H pylori* eradication at first ulcer recurrence; and (3) continuous maintenance therapy with a histamine2 receptor antagonist (ranitidine hydrochloride). Two *H pylori* eradication therapies were compared: classic triple therapy and omeprazole plus amoxicillin. Probabilities for ulcer recurrence are by meta-analysis of published randomized trials. Health care resources used in the management of duodenal ulcer recurrence were by expert physician panel. All **costs** are in 1993 Canadian dollars. RESULTS: Duodenal ulcer recurrence at 6 months (symptomatic and asymptomatic) with placebo was 65.4% and 12.8% with maintenance ranitidine therapy. Where eradication of *H pylori* was successful (85% of patients), the ulcer recurrence rate to 12 months was 3.7%. Treatment with ranitidine and triple therapy to eradicate *H pylori* on first presentation has an expected 1-year cost of $253 with 15 symptomatic recurrences per 100 patients; *H pylori* eradication by omeprazole plus amoxicillin had similar expected costs ($272) and outcomes (15 recurrences per 100 patients). Both of these early *H pylori* eradication strategies were dominant (less costly with same or better outcomes) over intermittent or continuous maintenance ranitidine therapy or delayed (after first recurrence) *H pylori* eradication. CONCLUSION: Our analysis provides **economic** evidence in support of the recent guidance that for persons with duodenal ulcer, early attempts to eradicate *H pylori* are recommended.

Publication Type Journal Article.

Textwords   Cost-effectiveness (title and abstract)
                                   Costs (abstract)
                                   Economic
                                   Decision analysis

REFERENCES

1. Drummond M. Evidence-based medicine and cost-effectiveness: uneasy bedfellows [EBM Note]. Evidence-Based Medicine 1998;3:133.
2. Elixhauser A, Halpern M, Schmier J, Luce BR. Health care CBA and CEA from 1991 to 1996: an updated bibliography. Med Care 1998;36(5 Suppl):MS1–9.
3. Schulman KA, Glick HA, Yabroff KR, Eisenberg JM. Introduction to clinical economics: assessment of cancer therapies. Monogr Natl Cancer Inst 1995;19:1–19.
4. O'Brien B. Principles of economic evaluation for health care programs. J Rheumatol 1995;22: 1399–402.
5. Covinsky KE, King JT Jr, Quinn LM, et al. Do acute care for elders units increase hospital costs? A cost analysis using the hospital perspective. J Am Geriatr Soc 1997;45:729–34.
6. Golaszewski T, Snow D, Lynch W, et al. A benefit-to-cost analysis of a work-site health promotion program. J Occup Med 1992;34:1164–72.
7. Salzmann P, Kerlikowske K, Phillips K. Cost-effectiveness of extending screening mammography guidelines to include women 40 to 49 years of age. Ann Intern Med 1997;127:955–65.
8. Glennie J. Technology overview: pharmaceuticals: pharmacoeconomic evaluations of clozapine in treatment-resistant schizophrenia and risperidone in chronic schizophrenia. Ottawa: Canadian Coordinating Office for Health Technology Assessment (CCOHTA): 1997 Jul.
9. Zarnke KB, Levine MA, O'Brien BJ. Cost-benefit analyses in the health care literature: don't judge a study by its label. J Clin Epidemiol 1997;50:813–22.
10. Rosenheck R, Cramer J, Weichun X, et al. A comparison of clozapine and haloperidol in hospitalized patients with refractory schizophrenia. N Engl J Med 1997;337:809–15.
11. Jones P. Commentary on "Clozapine reduced symptoms and side effects in patients who had refractory schizophrenia." Evidence-Based Mental Health 1998;1:82. [Comment on: Rosenheck R, Cramer J, Weichun X, et al. A comparison of clozapine and haloperidol in hospitalized patients with refractory schizophrenia. N Engl J Med 1997;337:809–15.]
12. Anis AH, Tugwell PX, Wells GA, Stewart DG. A cost effectiveness analysis of cyclosporine in rheumatoid arthritis. J Rheumatol 1996;23:609–16.
13. Lave JR, Frank RG, Schulberg HC, Kamlet MS. Cost-effectiveness of treatments for major depression in primary care practice. Arch Gen Psychiatry 1998;55:645–51.

9

Qualitative Studies

Susan Marks, BA, BEd

Up to this point, the study designs that we have described (for example, randomized controlled trial, cohort study, case-control study) have been what are called **quantitative** studies. Quantitative study designs are most appropriate when answering questions of "how many" or "how much." For example, if you want to find out whether guided imagery could reduce pain in children with leukemia, you should look for a randomized controlled trial in which children are randomly allocated to participate in interactive guided imagery sessions (experimental group) or to an equal amount of time simply visiting with a volunteer (control group). After each visit, the two groups are compared to see how many children in each group report reductions in pain. Some types of research or clinical questions, however, are best answered using another type of study design called **qualitative**. When you want to know about how people *feel* or *experience* certain situations, a qualitative study is usually a better choice. If you wanted to understand, for example, how the families of children diagnosed with cancer learned to cope with the diagnosis and the changes it brought to their lives, a qualitative study would be more likely to provide meaningful information. In such a study, a researcher might hold in-depth interviews with parents of children with cancer, beginning with a general statement, such as, "Tell me what it was like to find out that your child had cancer." The researcher would then systematically analyze verbatim transcripts of the interviews, looking for common themes and connections among them to describe the experience of parents coping with a child's diagnosis of cancer.

To better understand what qualitative research is all about, it may be helpful to see how it differs from quantitative research. The purpose of this comparison is not to determine which method is "better." Quantitative study designs have a long history in the health care literature, whereas qualitative studies are relatively new. Proponents of both quantitative and qualitative research continue to debate the relative merits and weaknesses of each, and often become entrenched in views that one or the other is more valid. For our purposes, we propose that both qualitative and quantitative studies have a place in health care research, and the most important thing is to look for the type of study design that can provide the best answers to your questions—and how we define "best" can also vary, according to the question asked.

Qualitative studies usually differ from quantitative studies in terms of the type of questions they address, how samples are chosen, methods of data collection and analysis, and how results are presented. These differences are summarized in Table 9–1, and some of the key points will be illustrated in the Clinical Example given in the next section.

CLINICAL EXAMPLE

Wilson[1] did a qualitative study to better understand the experiences of elderly people admitted to nursing homes on a planned or unplanned basis, and how they made the transition to nursing home life. Fifteen adults aged 76 to 97 years who were admitted to nursing homes participated in semi-structured 1-hour interviews during the first month after admission. Interviews began with broad questions, such as, "Can you tell me what is it like for you being in a nursing home?"

During the interviews, the researcher observed and made notes of the participants' nonverbal behavior (for example, facial expressions) and activities (for example, lying in bed). The interviews were tape recorded and transcribed verbatim. After the fifteenth person was interviewed, **data saturation** occurred—that is, no new understandings (for example, categories or themes) were arising from additional interviews—and no further interviews were done. Data from the interviews were analyzed using the **constant comparative method**. Concepts were identified based on data from the first interviews (for example, statements such as, "I get awful lonely and depressed" could be labeled as concepts of "feeling lonely" and "feeling depressed"); data from subsequent interviews were then compared to see if they could be labeled using the same concepts, or if they needed new ones (for example, a statement such as, "I'm afraid if I leave my room I'll get lost and won't find my way back" could be labeled as a new concept of "feeling afraid"). Similar concepts were then grouped together under unifying categories (for example, feeling lonely, feeling depressed, and feeling afraid could be grouped together under a category of "feeling overwhelmed." From this analysis, a theory emerged about the transition to nursing home life. Participants seemed to progress through three phases. During the first phase, the *overwhelmed phase*, participants cried, felt lonely, and longed to go home, but tried to hide these feelings from their families. During the second phase, the *adjustment phase*, participants began to think more positively about the future and everyday living, developed new social networks, and started to deal with such issues as the loss of control resulting from the nursing home rules and regulations. During the third phase, the *initial acceptance phase*, participants began to take action, making new friends and getting involved in activities, and felt more confident.

HOW A QUALITATIVE STUDY IS DONE

This example illustrates a number of the features common to many qualitative studies:

Table 9–1
Common Features of Qualitative and Quantitative Studies

Features	Qualitative Studies	Quantitative Studies
Type of question	Most appropriate for questions about *meaning* and how people *feel and experience* situations.	Most appropriate for questions of "how many" (patients get better) or "how much" (do they get better).
Sampling	*Theoretical* or *purposeful* sampling of a relatively small number of people who have in-depth knowledge or experience of the topic of interest. The goal is to learn about people in a specific context and not to generate findings that will be applicable to a wide variety of people. Although there may be few participants, there are many "sampling units" of textual data generated from each participant.	*Probability* sampling to ensure that the sample is representative of a more general population and to minimize bias. The goal is to ensure that the findings will be generalizable to general populations of people. Large sample sizes are often needed to detect differences between groups.
Data collection	Data collection often involves *unstructured interviews* although other methods are also used (for example, observation of people in natural settings and focus groups). Responses given in interviews with the first few participants may lead to modifications in how later interviews are conducted (iterative approach).	Systematic data collection using *structured formats. Blinding* of data collectors or participants is some-times necessary to avoid biasing results.
Analysis	Data analysis takes place *concurrent with data collection* process, and is ongoing. Units of analysis are *thoughts or concepts*, which are classified into categories or themes.	Date analysis takes place *after all data are collected.* Units of analysis are *numbers*, which are combined and manipulated using statistical tests.
Presentation of findings	Rich, detailed findings are presented in *narrative format*, sometimes accompanied by diagrams of theoretical models. Many direct quotations of participants are included.	Findings pertaining to the sample or specific subsamples are summarized in terms of **numerical relations** or **statistics**.

- The **research question** focused on the experiences of a particular group of people in a particular context (that is, how elderly people experienced the transition to nursing home life).

- Selection of the **study sample** was *theoretical* or *purposeful*. The intent was to select the participants best able to meet the informational needs of the study.[2] Therefore, it was more important to select a small number of participants with in-depth knowledge of the study topic than to select a large number randomly. The sample size was not identified ahead of time, but was determined by the ongoing process of data collection and analysis. Data collection stopped after the fifteenth interview because no new themes emerged during it (data saturation occurred). This highlights the **iterative approach** that is often used in qualitative studies. Data collection and analysis occur concurrently, and influence the next step of the research process. For example, immediately after the interview with the first participant, the researcher will analyze the data, beginning with the identification and classification of words and thoughts into common themes and categories. This analysis may lead the researcher to slightly modify the questions that she poses to the second participant. Similarly, after the second interview, the researcher examines the data to see what fits and does not fit into themes or categories identified from the first interview, and whether additional refinements or categories are warranted. This process continues until data saturation occurs.

    In the example, data were collected using different methods and sources. Although the interview transcripts were the primary data source, field notes made by the researcher provided additional, complementary data on participants' non-verbal behaviors and activity levels.

- The **unit of analysis** was words or concepts, rather than numbers as in quantitative studies. Data were analyzed using the *constant comparative method*. The interview transcripts and field notes from the first interview were analyzed line by line to identify underlying concepts. Data from the second interview were then compared to see if they could be labeled using these same concepts, or whether new concepts were needed. As this process continued with subsequent interviews, similar concepts were grouped together to form categories; and through the integration of categories, a theory was developed.[3]

- The **study findings** were presented in a narrative format, with numerous examples of *verbatim statements* made by participants. For example, to illustrate some of the aspects of the initial *overwhelmed* phase, the following quotation was reported: "I get awful lonely and depressed. I forget a lot of things, my mind isn't working the way it should... I don't want to be a burden to my daughter and her husband." These examples help the reader to see how the researcher arrived at certain themes. In some cases, the researcher may develop a model or theory that attempts to explain processes or how different themes are interrelated.

    Reports of qualitative studies can be quite lengthy, restricted only by the word limits of the publishing journal. Indeed, many authors of qualitative reports find it difficult to convey the depth and richness of the data they have collected in the limited space available in most journals. Similarly, the above summary is only a superficial description of Wilson's findings to give readers the flavor of qualitative research.

TYPES OF QUALITATIVE STUDIES

Just as there are different types of quantitative study designs, there are also a number of different qualitative designs that are defined according to the underlying theoretical framework or the data collection and analysis methods. Types of qualitative studies or methods include grounded theory, ethnography, focus groups, and participant and nonparticipant observation. As well, the results of multiple qualitative studies on a specific topic can be combined and analyzed in a systematic review (sometimes called a **meta-ethnography**, **meta-synthesis**, or even **meta-analysis**). The nature of the analysis is, however, obviously different from that used in quantitative systematic reviews and meta-analyses. Three of the more common types of qualitative research found in the literature—phenomenology, grounded theory, and ethnography—will be described briefly. These three qualitative methods aim to describe the complexity of human experiences in context.[4]

Phenomenology is concerned with describing the human or "lived" experience using the subjective or first-person experience as a source of knowledge. It is often used when little is known about a topic.[5] Gravelle[6] did a phenomenological study to describe parents' day-to-day experiences of managing their child's chronic, life-threatening, progressive illness. Eleven parents with eight children who had conditions such as muscular dystrophy and cerebral palsy participated in unstructured interviews. The parents reported successive challenges because of the progressive nature of the diseases, and experienced cycles of defining adversity and managing adversity with each new challenge. Defining adversity was shaped by specific features of the child's condition (for example, rate of disease progression), family characteristics (for example, degree of parents' acceptance of the condition), and the magnitude of the specific challenge (for example, adapting to being confined to a wheel chair). Managing adversity involved seeking information, services, and equipment; planning and preparing for the future; negotiating special services and free time; and arranging resources.

Grounded theory studies are designed, as the name suggests, to develop theory grounded in the real world of the participants. Thus, in addition to describing phenomena, grounded theory studies attempt to explain them.[3] The study by Wilson[1] on how elderly people adapted to nursing home life is an example of grounded theory. Another good example is a study by Schreiber[7] on the process of women's recovery from depression. Twenty women who had recovered from depression participated in interviews lasting about 90 minutes. Interview transcripts were analyzed using constant comparative analysis. A theory emerged that explained the six-stage process of "(re)defining my self" that the women went through as they recovered from depression.

Ethnographic studies seek to learn about how people interpret their experience and adapt their behavior within the context of their own culturally defined environment.[8] A good example is a study done by Tourigny[9] involving six African-American youths who had deliberately exposed themselves to HIV. All of the participants were HIV positive, and had at least one family member with HIV infection or AIDS. Tourigny met with these youths over time, with meetings often taking place in the respondents' homes while they carried on with activities such as washing dishes, caring for family members, or keeping watch over gang-related traffic in the neighborhoods. The stories of each of the youths and why they deliberately sought exposure to HIV were presented in a narrative format, with many direct quotes. For example, Brendon's story began as follows:

> Brandon was 22 when we met. A man of courtly manners and a gentle presence, he would cry at any mention of his 40-year-old sister, Debra—her illness, her sex work, her drug habit, and, particularly her children: his niece, a healthy 8-year-old, and his 5-year-old AIDS-afflicted nephew. {....} After more than 3 years of unemployment, friendships with people who are still working gradually offered little but embarrassment. His own despair eroded his emotional resilience; his easy smile became frozen, and he started talking about wanting to die. One hot afternoon, Brendon looked over my shoulder as he said,
>
> "Yo...doc, I got it too. Everybody was raggin me about not getting nowhere, not getting no job, not doing nothing. Well there ain't nothing to do here. I looked at my sister, and she got everybody seeing to her hand and foot and she ain't even sick. This AIDS things don't need make you sick at all, but people sure listen up when you talk. She's getting good money from the feds..." (page 155)

Tournigy interpreted these stories in the context of the social inequalities of inner city life. She found that the youths were overwhelmed by worry, depression, caregiving, and hopelessness, and robbed of their childhood by poverty. They were deeply involved with their loved ones, so leaving was not an alternative. With no other obvious recourse, AIDS offered a way to access care and resources.

SUMMARY

Qualitative studies generally differ from quantitative studies such as randomized controlled trials or cohort studies, in terms of the type of question asked, sample selection, data collection and analysis, and reporting of results. Qualitative studies provide the most relevant information when you want to know how people feel or experience certain situations. The number of people sampled is usually much smaller than for quantitative studies, and participants are often selected on the basis of their knowledge or experience of the content area. Common methods of data collection include in-depth unstructured interviews, focus groups, observation, and use of print records, such as diaries or historical accounts. Whereas the unit of analysis in quantitative studies is primarily numbers, the unit of analysis in qualitative studies is a thought or a concept. Study findings are presented in the form of rich, detailed narratives that describe common themes and understandings, or sometimes as diagrams that depict how different themes are interrelated.

SEARCHING FOR QUALITATIVE STUDIES

There has been some debate about how to assess the quality of qualitative studies. Indeed, some believe that the very nature of qualitative research precludes the type of objective assessment that is applied to quantitative research. (This argument arises from an underlying belief that truth is subjective and inextricably tied to context, thereby making it inappropriate to apply objective assessment criteria.) Others have attempted to identify potential criteria for appraising qualitative studies.[3,10–13] Some of these criteria are general in nature, and could apply to either qualitative or quantitative studies (for example, is there a clear statement of the question; is a qualitative design appropriate to answer this question; is the process for selecting participants clearly described; are the participants described in sufficient detail to enable you to judge the extent to which the findings will be "transferable" or "generalizable" to other groups of people?).

Because of this lack of agreement about how to assess the quality of qualitative studies, and because of their relative newness to the health care literature, no methodological HEDGES have been developed to help readers to identify only studies of the highest quality. In fact, relatively few index terms are defined in MEDLINE that relate to qualitative research, and none in EMBASE. On the other hand, CINAHL has many index terms relating to the various types of qualitative study designs.

CINAHL Database of Nursing and Allied Health Literature

Index Terms and Textwords for Qualitative Studies

Index terms
Qualitative studies
Ethnological research
Ethnonursing research
Focus groups
Grounded theory
Phenomenological research
Qualitative validity
    Confirmability (research)
    Credibility (research)
    Dependability (research)
    Transferability
Purposive sample
Theoretical sample
Phenomenology
Ethnography
Observational methods
    Nonparticipant observation
    Participant observation
Life experiences

Textwords

Colaizzi:	Lived experience
Constant compar:	Merleau:
Emic	Narrative analysis

Ethnon:	Participant observ:
Etic	Phenomenolog:
Focus group	Qualitative
Giorgi:	Ricoeur
Grounded theory	Spiegelberg:
Heidegger:	Theoretical samp:
Hermeneutic	Van kaam:
Husserl:	Van Manen

All extracts from the CINAHL® Thesaurus Copyright © 1999, Cinahl Information Systems. Reprinted with permission from Cinahl Information Systems.

MEDLINE

MeSH, and Textwords for Qualitative Studies

MeSH
Nursing methodology research

Text words
Qualitative research
Ethnon:
Emic
Etic
Ethnograph:
Hermeneutic:
Heidegger:
Husserl:
Colaizzi:
Giorgi:
Van kaam:
Van Manen
Participant observ:
Constant compar:
Focus group:
Grounded theory
Narrative analysis
Lived experience
Life experience:
Theoretical samp:

Do not search using the textword "phenomenolog:" in MEDLINE. Many articles in MEDLINE use the term "phenomenology" to mean the description or classification of things, and not to refer to the qualitative design or methodology of phenomenology.

PsycINFO

Only one index term is available in PsycINFO for qualitative studies: ethnography. Use the textwords from CINAHL and MEDLINE for retrievals.

EMBASE/EXCERPTA MEDICA

No high quality terms are available in EMBASE/Excerpta Medica for retrieval of qualitative studies. Use the textwords from CINAHL and MEDLINE for retrievals.

EXAMPLES

Example 9–1
Phenomenology
Herth K. Integrating hearing loss into one's life. Qual Health Res 1998;8:207–23.

In this phenomenological study. Herth sought to better understand the experiences of people with a hearing loss as they tried to integrate the loss into their everyday lives. Thirty-two people were recruited from churches and physician's offices and all had a hearing loss that they felt interfered with their communication with others. Semi-structured interviews were done, usually in the participant's home. Questions included what the hearing loss meant to the person, how it affected their everyday lives, things they had to change because of the hearing loss, and what they believed would happen in the future. Analysis of the interview transcripts identified a number of common themes; 6 of the participants were interviewed a second time to confirm the themes that the author identified. The underlying theme was one of *dancing with*, which reflected the ongoing process of adjustment involved in integrating the hearing loss into one's life. The theme of *dancing with loss and fear* involved a loss of feeling capable, loss of control and independence, loss of connectedness or belonging, loss of dignity, and loss of self esteem. The sense of loss was accompanied by fear—fear of failure, fear of dependency, fear of ridicule, fear of being slighted, fear of new situations, fear of people and chance encounters, and fear of sudden noises. The theme of *dancing with fluctuating feelings* reflected the "emotional roller coaster ride" of trying to integrate the hearing loss into one's life. Sometimes one feeling dominated, whereas at other times, several feelings occurred concurrently. These feelings included grief, anger, denial, frustration, isolation, depression, loneliness, inadequacy, sadness, sorrow, discouragement, distress, and uncertainty. The theme of *dancing with courage amidst change* reflected the need to deal with the unwanted and unexpected changes that resulted from the hearing loss. The changes involved doing things differently, planning things in advance, and generally exerting a great amount of energy when expressing themselves and listening to others. Many of the participants showed courage and resilience in dealing with these changes and moving ahead with their lives. The theme of *dancing with an altered life perspective* reflected how participants changed their life perspective in response to the losses and changes that they

CINAHL Record for Example 9–1

Accession Number   1998043845.

Authors   Herth K.

Institution   Department of Nursing, Georgia Southern University, PO Box 8158, Statesboro, GA 30480-8158.

Title   Integrating hearing loss into one's life.

Source   Qualitative Health Research. 8(2): 207–23, 1998 Mar. (51 ref)

CINAHL Subject Headings
* Adaptation Psychological
Adolescence
Adult
Age of Onset
Aged
Aged, 80 and Over
Audiorecording
Confirmability (Research)
Convenience Sample
Credibility (Research)

Dependability (Research)
Fear
Hearing Disorders/nu [Nursing]
*Hearing Disorder/pf [Psychosocial Factors]
*Life Change Events
Middle Age
Personal Loss
Phenomenological Research
Semi-Structured Interview
Thematic Analysis
Transferability

Abstract
Hearing loss is the single most prevalent chronic physical disability in the United States. Little is known about the experience of integrating hearing loss as a part of one's life, particularly from the perspective of the hearing-impaired person. This **phenomenolog**ical inquiry explored how adults with onset of hearing loss after acquisition of language integrate the hearing loss into their lives. The author interviewed 32 deafened adults. Using a modification of P.F. **Colaizzi's** method of data analysis, four distinct themes, each with subthemes, emerged around a core variable labeled as dancing with. These themes were dancing with loss and fear, dancing with fluctuating feelings, dancing with courage amidst change, and dancing with an altered life perspective. This study provides a beginning understanding of how people integrate a hearing loss into their lives and is the first step in developing and implementing appropriate strategies to provide assistance to others experiencing hearing loss. (51 ref)

Publication Type   Journal Article. Research. Tables/Charts.

experienced. They tried to gain control of their lives by seeking support and information, developing new problem solving skills and risk taking behaviors, implementing new approaches, using humor, and finding hope and meaning in their hearing loss.

Retrieval Can Be Done Using Any of the Following:

CINAHL indexing	Confirmability (research)
	Credibility (research)
	Dependability (research)
	Phenomenological research
	Thematic analysis
	Transferability
Textwords	Phenomenol: (abstract)
	Colaizzi: (abstract)

This citation is not found in MEDLINE at this time. Only a few articles from 1993 are indexed for the journal *Qualitative Health Research.*

Example 9–2
Grounded theory
D'Auria JP, Christian BJ, Richardson LF. Through the looking glass: children's perceptions of growing up with cystic fibrosis. Can J Nurs Res 1997;29:99–112.

D'Auria and colleagues were interested in children's experiences of growing up with a chronic disease, cystic fibrosis. Using a grounded theory approach, they conducted a study of 20 children aged 6 to 12 years who had been diagnosed with cystic fibrosis by age 3. In 30 to 60 minute interviews, children were asked to visualize their experiences of growing up with cystic fibrosis and to give advice to children who were newly diagnosed with the disease. The interview transcripts, supplemented with field notes taken by the interviewer, were analyzed using the constant comparative method. The experience of growing up with cystic fibrosis seemed to focus on the central phenomena of *discovering a sense of difference.* Four main themes emerged from the children's accounts. The first, *puzzling out the meaning,* referred to children's memories of finding out from their mothers that they had cystic fibrosis and their surprise at realizing that they were not like other children. For most children, the discovery of these differences began when they entered school and began to interact with a peer group. The second theme, *being picked on and teased,* described children's experiences of stress and learning to cope with negative peer responses to their visible differences, particularly at a time when peer acceptance was crucial. In time, the children learned to think of themselves as 'normal' and to be less affected by the reactions of other children. The third theme, *telling others,* had to do with the particular characteristics of cystic fibrosis that called the most attention to their differences, that is, coughing and taking medicine. To avoid having to explain these differences to their peers, they tried to control how others viewed them by keeping secrets and selectively disclosing information about their illness to friends they considered trustworthy. The fourth theme, *keeping up*, reflected the physical and functional limitations imposed by cystic fibrosis (for example, not having the energy to run as fast as other children) and how these limitations made it difficult to fit in and compete with their peers. Some of the children withdrew, which further reduced their opportunities to fit in, whereas others learned to pace themselves so that they could control their symptoms.

Retrieval Can Be Done Using Any of the Following:

CINAHL indexing	Constant comparative method
	Grounded theory
	Purposive sample
	Qualitative studies
	Thematic analysis
Textwords	Qualitative (abstract)
	Grounded theory (abstract)
	Purposive sample (abstract)
MEDLINE indexing	Nursing methodology research
Textwords	Qualitative (abstract)
	Grounded theory (abstract)
	Purposive sample (abstract)

Example 9–3

Ethnography

Anderson NLR. Decisions about substance abuse among adolescents in juvenile detention. Image J Nurs Sch 1996;28:65–70.

Anderson did an ethnographic study involving 20 adolescent girls in a juvenile detention facility to learn about how they made decisions to stop abusing substances and to explore the dynamics of interaction among these young women. Data were collected during 6 focus groups, each involving 2 to 3 adolescents; participant observation during daily activities and events; and individual interviews. Content analysis of the focus group transcripts revealed that the adolescents made decisions about future abstinence based in part on the dynamic interactions with other adolescents during their detention. Four categories for making resolutions about future abstinence emerged. *Recreating past experience* involved remembering the past and sharing similar experiences about things like difficulties at home, peer pressure, specific incidents of substance abuse, and the consequences of these incidents. *Planning resolutions* to maintain abstinence arose from fear and the desire to put their lives in order for the future. The teens discussed future plans and encouraged each other to have faith in themselves. In

CINAHL Record for Example 9–2

Accession Number   1998033295.

Authors   D'Auria JP, Christian BJ, Richardson LF.

Institution   School of Nursing, University of North Carolina at Chapel Hill, CB #7460, Carrington Hall, Chapel Hill, NC 27599-7460. E-mail: jdauria.uncson@mhs.unc.edu.

Title   Through the looking glass: children's perceptions of growing up with cystic fibrosis.

Source   Canadian Journal of Nursing Research. 29(4):99–112, 1997 Winter. (41 ref)

CINAHL Subject Headings

Audiorecording	**Grounded Theory**
Child	Interviews
Coding	**Purposive Sample**
Constant Comparative Method	**Qualitative Studies**
*Cystic Fibrosis/pf [Psychosocial Factors]	Southeastern United States
Field Notes	**Thematic Analysis**
Funding Source	

Abstract
This **qualitative** study used a **grounded theory** approach to explore the unfolding of the chronic illness experience for children during middle childhood. A **purposive sample** of 20 children (6–12 years) with cystic fibrosis (CF) were interviewed. Discovering a sense of difference was found to be the central phenomenon that described the experience of having CF during the middle childhood years. Four central themes emerged in the stories of these children: (a) puzzling out the diagnosis, (b) being teased and picked on, (c) telling others, and (d) keeping up. The study concluded that interventions must focus on the psychosocial demands made on children with CF along their course of development. By designing interventions around meaningful outcomes in their daily lives, we will help children with CF find ways to feel normal while adhering to treatment regimens, thereby helping improve the quality of their lives. (41 ref)

Publication Type   Journal Article. Research.

MEDLINE Record for Example 9–2

Unique Identifier   98362777

Authors   D'Auria JP, Christian BJ, Richardson LF.

Institution   School of Nursing, University of North Carolina at Chapel Hill, USA. jdauria.uncson@mhs.unc.edu

Title   Through the looking glass: children's perceptions of growing up with cystic fibrosis.

Source   Can J Nurs Res 1997 Winter;29(4):99–112.

MeSH Subject Headings

*Adaptation Psychological	Male
*Attitude to Health	**Nursing Methodology Research**
Child	Peer Group
*Child Psychology	Questionnaires
Chronic Disease	*Self Concept
Cystic Fibrosis/*psychology	Social Behavior
Female	Support, U.S. Gov't, P.H.S.
Human	

Abstract
This **qualitative** study used a **grounded theory** approach to explore the unfolding of the chronic illness experience for children during middle childhood. A **purposive sample** of 20 children (6–12 years) with cystic fibrosis (CF) were interviewed. Discovering a sense of difference was found to be the central phenomenon that described the experience of having CF during the middle childhood years. Four central themes emerged in the stories of these children: (a) puzzling out the diagnosis, (b) being teased and picked on, (c) telling others, and (d) keeping up. The study concluded that interventions must focus on the psychosocial demands made on children with CF along their course of development. By designing interventions around meaningful outcomes in their daily lives, we will help children with CF find ways to feel normal while adhering to treatment regimens, thereby helping to improve the quality of their lives.

Publication Type   Journal Article

Permission to use abstract given by Journal.

CINAHL Record for Example 9-3

Accession Number   1996014845

NLM Unique Identifier   97063799

Authors   Anderson NLR.

Institution   UCLA School of Nursing, 10833 Le Conte Ave, Factor 5-234, Los Angeles, CA 90095-6919.

Title   Decisions about substance abuse among adolescents in juvenile detention.

Source   Image—The Journal of Nursing Scholarship. 28(1):65–70, 1996 Spring. (30 ref)

CINAHL Subject Headings

Adolescence
*Adolescent Psychology
Audiorecording
Content Analysis
Convenience Sample
*Decision Making
Ethnographic Research
Female
Field Notes

Focus Groups
Funding Source
Interviews
Participant Observation
*Prisoners
Problem Solving
Qualitative Studies
*Substance Abuse

Abstract
Ethnographic research was done to discover how adolescents make decisions about substance abuse while in juvenile detention. Segments of transcribed data from small focus group discussions portray the perspectives of 20 teenage girls in one juvenile detention facility located in a large metropolitan area. Observations and individual interviews corroborated the dynamic interactive dialogue among the teens during group discussions. The young women described the situations and problems that led to substance abuse and their subsequent detention. The sharing of life experiences provided an opportunity to reinforce resolutions to change and plans to abstain from troublesome behaviors in the future. (30 ref)

Publication Type   Journal Article.

MEDLINE Record for Example 9–3

Unique Identifier   97063799

Authors   Anderson NL

Address   UCLA Nursing, Los Angeles, USA.

Title   Decisions about substance abuse among adolescents in juvenile detention.

Source   Image J Nurs Sch 1996 Spring 28(1):65–70

MeSH Subject Headings

Adolescence

Adolescent Behavior

Adolescent, Institutionalized/
  *psychology

Anthropology, Cultural

Female

Focus Groups

Human

Juvenile Delinquency/*psychology

Peer Group

Substance-Related Disorders/
  prevention and control/*psychology

Support, Non-U.S. Gov't

Abstract

Ethnographic research was done to discover how adolescents make decisions about substance abuse while in juvenile detention. Segments of transcribed data from small focus group discussions portray the perspectives of 20 teenage girls in one juvenile detention facility located in a large metropolitan area. Observations and individual interviews corroborated the dynamic interactive dialogue occurring among the teens during group discussions. The young women described the situations and problems that led to substance abuse and their subsequent detention. The sharing of life experiences provided an opportunity to reinforce resolutions to change and plans to abstain from troublesome behaviors in the future.

Publication Type   Journal Article

considering reservations about resolutions, participants expressed concern about the future and the temptations they would have to confront when they left detention and went back to their home neighborhoods (for example, peer pressure to begin using substances again). As they expressed these concerns, the participants began *reinforcing both their own and each others resolutions.*

Retrieval Can Be Done Using Any of the Following

CINAHL index terms	Ethnographic research
	Focus groups
	Participant observation
	Qualitative studies
	Ethnographic research (abstract)
Textwords	Focus group (abstract)
MEDLINE index terms	None
Textwords	Ethnograph research (abstract)
	Focus group (abstract)

ASSIGNMENT

1. Often, people with disabilities require public health care services to assist them with various self-care activities (for example, bathing) or other activities of daily living. How do people with disabilities experience the care that they receive?
2. How do adult children come to deal with the anticipated death of their parents?
3. What role does culture play in the sexual attitudes and behavior of Latina adolescents?
4. Are there any studies that synthesize the findings of different studies of the experience of living with diabetes?

REFERENCES

1. Wilson SA. The transition to nursing home life: a comparison of planned and unplanned admissions. J Adv Nurs 1997;26:864–71.
2. Morse JM. Strategies for sampling. In: Morse JM, editor. Qualitative nursing research: a contemporary dialogue. Newbury Park (CA): Sage Publications; 1991. p. 127–45.
3. Corbin J, Strauss A. Grounded theory research: procedures, canons, and evaluative criteria. Qual Sociol 1990;13:3–21.
4. Lipson JC. The use of self in ethnographic research. In: Morse JM, editor. Qualitative nursing research: a contemporary dialogue. Newbury Park (CA): Sage Publications; 1991. p. 73–89.
5. Smith BA. The problem drinker's lived experience of suffering: an exploration using hermeneutic phenomenology. J Adv Nurs Sci 1998;27:213–22.
6. Gravelle AM. Caring for a child with a progressive illness during the complex chronic phase: parents' experience of facing adversity. J Adv Nurs 1997;25:738–45.
7. Schreiber R. (Re) defining my self: women's process of recovery from depression. Qual Health Res 1996;6:469–91.

8. Aamodt AM. Ethnography and epistemology: generating nursing knowledge In: Morse JM, editor. Qualitative nursing research: a contemporary dialogue. Newbury Park (CA): Sage Publications; 1991. p. 40–53.

9. Tourigny SC. Some new dying trick: African-American youths "choosing" HIV/AIDS. Qual Health Res 1998;8:149–67.

10. Elder NC, Miller WL. Reading and evaluating qualitative research. J Fam Pract 1995;41: 279–85.

11. Estabrooks CA. What kind of evidence does qualitative research offer cardiovascular nurses? Can J Cardiovascular Nursing 1997;8:31–4.

12. Forchuk C, Roberts J. How to critique qualitative research articles. Can J Nurs Res 1993;25: 47–55.

13. Greenlaugh T, Taylor R. How to read a paper: papers that go beyond numbers (qualitative research). BMJ 1997;315:740–3.

Appendix

FURTHER READING

JAMA Series on Evidence-Based Medicine

Guyatt GH, Rennie D. Users' guides to the medical literature [editorial]. JAMA 1993;270:2096–7.

Oxman AD, Sackett DL, Guyatt GH for the Evidence-Based Medicine Working Group. Users' guides to the medical literature. I. How to get started. JAMA 1993;270:2093–7.

Guyatt GH, Sackett DL, Cook DJ for the Evidence-Based Medicine Working Group. Users' guides to the medical literature. II. How to use an article about therapy or prevention. A. Are the results of the study valid? JAMA 1993;270:2598–601.

Guyatt GH, Sackett DL, Cook DJ for the Evidence-Based Medicine Working Group. Users' guides to the medical literature. II. How to use an article about therapy or prevention. B. What were the results and will they help me in caring for my patients? JAMA 1994;271:59–63.

Jaeschke R, Guyatt GH, Sackett DL for the Evidence-Based Medicine Working Group. Users' guides to the medical literature. III. How to use an article about a diagnostic test. A. Are the results of the study valid? JAMA 1994;271:389–91.

Jaeschke R, Guyatt GH, Sackett DL for the Evidence-Based Medicine Working Group. Users' guides to the medical literature. III. How to use an article about a diagnostic test. B. What are the results and will they help me in caring for my patients? JAMA 1994;271:703–7.

Levine M, Walter S, Lee H, Haines T, et al. for the Evidence-Based Medicine Working Group. Users' guides to the medical literature. IV. How to use an article about harm. JAMA 1994;271:1615–9.

Laupacis A, Wells G, Richardson S, Tugwell P for the Evidence-Based Medicine Working Group. Users' guides to the medical literature. V. How to use an article about prognosis. JAMA 1994;272:234–7.

Oxman AD, Cook DL, Guyatt GH for the Evidence-Based Medicine Working Group. Users' guides to the medical literature. VI. How to use an overview. JAMA 1994;272:1367–71.

Richardson WS, Detsky AS for the Evidence-Based Medicine Working Group. Users' guides to the medical literature. VII. How to use a clinical decision analysis. A. Are the results of the study valid? JAMA 1995;273:1292–5.

Richardson WS, Detsky AS for the Evidence-Based Medicine Working Group. Users' guides to the medical literature. VII. How to use a clinical decision analysis. B. What are the results and will they help me in caring for my patients? JAMA 1995;273:1610–3.

Hayward RSA, Wilson MC, Tunis SR, et al for the Evidence-Based Medicine Working Group. Users' guides to the medical literature. VIII. How to use clinical practice guidelines. A. Are the recommendations valid? JAMA 1995;274:570–4.

Wilson MC, Hayward RSA, Tunis SR, et al. for the Evidence-Based Medicine Working Group. Users' guides to the medical literature. VIII. How to use clinical practice guidelines. B. What are the recommendations and will they help you in caring for your patients? JAMA 1995;274: 1630–2.

Guyatt GH, Sackett DL, Sinclair JC, et al. for the Evidence-Based Medicine Working Group. Users' guides to the medical literature. IX. A method for grading health care recommendations. JAMA 1995;274:1800–4.

Naylor CD, Guyatt GH for the Evidence-Based Medicine Working Group. Users' guides to the medical literature. X. How to use an article reporting variations in the outcomes of health services. JAMA 1996;275:554–8.

Naylor CD, Guyatt GH for the Evidence-Based Medicine Working Group. Users' guides to the medical literature. XI. How to use an article about a clinical utilization review. JAMA 1996;275: 1435–9.

Guyatt GH, Naylor CD, Juniper E, et al. for the Evidence-Based Medicine Working Group. Users' guides to the medical literature. XII. How to use articles about health-related quality of life. JAMA 1997;277:1232–7.

Drummond MF, Richardson WS, O'Brien BJ, et al. for the Evidence-Based Medicine Working Group. Users' guides to the medical literature. XIII. How to use an article on economic analysis of clinical practice. A. Are the results of the study valid? JAMA 1997;277:1552–7.

O'Brien BJ, Heyland D, Richardson WS, et al. for the Evidence-Based Medicine Working Group. Users' guides to the medical literature. XIII. How to use an article on economic analysis of clinical practice. B. What are the results and will they help me in caring for my patients? JAMA 1997;277:1802–6.

Sackett DL. On some clinically useful measures of the effects of treatment [editorial]. Evidence Based Medicine 1996;1:37–8.

Altman DG. Use of confidence intervals to indicate uncertainty in research findings [editorial]. Evidence Based Medicine 1996;1:101–2.

Sackett DL, Deeks JJ, Altman DG. Down with odds ratios! [editorial]. Evidence Based Medicine 1996;1:164–6.

Jadad AR, Gagliardi A. Rating health information on the Internet: navigating to knowledge or Babel? JAMA 1998;279:611–4.

Other editorials from *ACP Journal Club* and *Evidence-based Medicine*.

ANNALS OF INTERNAL MEDICINE SERIES ON SYSTEMATIC REVIEWS

Mulrow C, Cook DJ, Davidoff F. Systematic reviews: critical links in the great chain of evidence [editorial]. Ann Intern Med 1997;126:389–91.

Cook DJ, Mulrow CD, Haynes RB. Systematic reviews: synthesis of best evidence for clinical decisions. Ann Intern Med 1997;126:376–80.

Hunt DL, McKibbon A. Locating and appraising systematic reviews. Ann Intern Med 1997;126:532–8. http://www.acponline.org/journals/annals/01apr97/systemat.htm

McQuay HJ, Moore, RA. Using numerical results from systematic reviews in clinical practice. Ann Intern Med 1997;126:712–20.

Badget RG, O'Keefe MO, Henderson MC. Using systematic reviews in clinical education. Ann Intern Med 1997;126:886–91.

Bero LA, Jadad AR. How consumers and policy makers can use systematic reviews for decision making. Ann Intern Med 1997;127:37–42.

Counsell C. Formulating questions and locating primary studies for inclusion in systematic reviews. Ann Intern Med 1997;127:380–7.

Meade MO, Richardson WS. Selecting and appraising studies for a systematic review. Ann Intern Med 1997;127:531–7.

Cook DJ, Greengold NL, Ellrodt AG, Weingarten SR. The relation between systematic reviews and practice guidelines. Ann Intern Med 1997;127:210–6.

Lau J, Ioannidis JPA, Schmid CH. Quantitative synthesis in systematic reviews. Ann Intern Med 1997;127:820–6.

Mulrow C, Langhorne P, Grimshaw J. Integrating heterogeneous pieces of evidence in systematic reviews. Ann Intern Med 1997;127:989–95.

EVIDENCE-BASED HEALTH CARE INTERNET RESOURCES

What it is and isn't

http://cebm.jr2.ox.ac.uk/ebmisisnt.html

http://www.ohsu.edu/bicc-informatics/ebm/

http://hiru.mcmaster.ca/ebm/userguid/overview.htm

Other good sources

http://www.mssm.edu/library/resources/ebm.htm

http://www.shef.ac.uk/uni/academic/R-Z/scharr/ir/netting.html

http://www.amda.ab.ca/cpgs/frm_main.htm (practice guidelines)

http://www.cma.ca/cpgs/ (practice guidelines)

http://www.guidelines.gov/ (practice guidelines)

EBHC organizations

http://www.ohsu.edu/bicc-informatics/ebm/ebm_org.htm

http://cebm.jr2.ox.ac.uk/

Cochrane

http://hiru.mcmaster.ca/COCHRANE/DEFAULT.HTM

TIPS FOR ONLINE DATABASE COMPREHENSIVE SEARCHING

1. Use multiple bibliographic databases (MEDLINE, CINAHL, EMBASE/Excerpta Medica, and PsycINFO will cover most of the main stream health care literature).

2. Use databases of different kinds (e.g., citation, theses, research, PubMed "related articles" feature).

3. Extend the years of searching.

4. Have more than one set of searchers do your main searching independently—each searcher will retrieve relevant, unique citations.

5. Find out how the articles that you already have are indexed and work backwards using the index terms from the original articles. Bibliographies and personal files are often good places to find relevant citations to start with.

6. Avoid major emphasis (starring).

7. Avoid, or use AND NOT carefully. You can NOT out what you are truly interested in.

8. Avoid subheadings—use other methods of limiting information.

9. Make sure you are using all the explodes that are possible **AND** make sense.

10. Make sure you know the definitions of the terms you are using e.g., in MEDLINE adults are anyone who is from 19 to 44 years old—anyone over the age of 45 is considered to be middle aged.

11. Remember the "specificity" rule in constructing strategies (e.g., definition of "nutrition" may need many terms or groupings of terms [vitamin deficiency, protein restriction, and so on]).

12. Use a combination of textwords and index words.

13. For textwords make sure you remember
    alternative spellings (randomized and randomised)
    differences in terminology across disciplines (bed sores and decubitus ulcers)
    differences in terminology across national boundaries (SIDS and cot death)
    differences in historical naming (unwed mothers, *Camplybacter pylori*).
    short forms for terms (AIDS and acquired immunodeficiency syndrome)
    brand and generic names (Viagra and sildenafil)

14. Make sure you use terms that are somewhat related (mortality and survival analysis).

15. Use author searching, study names (GISSI, GUSTO, SOLVD), locations (Mayo clinic), manufacturers of drugs or products.

16. Search using opposites for some topics (e.g. if you are interested in "tallness" make sure you search for being "short" too.

Golden rule of searching
Keep track of what you have done!!!

Index